W9-BXY-627

The
Epidemiological
Approach

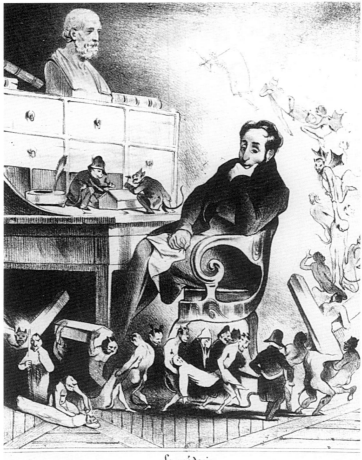

Le médecin,

Pourquoi, diable! mes malades s'en vont ils donc tous? .... j'ai beau les saig
les purger, les droguer .... je n'y comprends rien!

Honoré Daumier (1808–1879). THE DOCTOR: 'How the devil does it happen that all my
patients succumb? ... Yet I bleed them, I physic them, I drug them ... I simply can't understand!'
(Reproduced courtesy of the Bibliothèque Nationale de France)

The Epidemiological Approach

An Introduction to Epidemiology in Medicine

Fourth edition

Nicholas J Wald

Centre for Environmental and Preventive Medicine
Wolfson Institute of Preventive Medicine
Charterhouse Square
London EC1M 6BQ

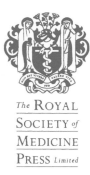

The ROYAL
SOCIETY *of*
MEDICINE
PRESS *Limited*

**WOLFSON INSTITUTE
OF PREVENTIVE
MEDICINE**

© 1988, 1991, 1996, 2004 Nicholas J Wald

Published jointly by

Wolfson Institute of Preventive Medicine
Charterhouse Square, London EC1M 6BQ, UK

Royal Society of Medicine Press Ltd
1 Wimpole Street, London W1G 0AE, UK
Tel: +44 (0)20 7290 2921
Fax: +44 (0)20 7290 2929
E-mail: publishing@rsm.ac.uk
Website: www.rsmpress.co.uk

Previous editions published by the Wolfson Institute of Preventive Medicine

Fourth edition 2004

Apart from any fair dealing for the purposes of research or private study, criticism or review, as permitted under the UK Copyright, Designs and Patents Act, 1988, no part of this publication may be reproduced, stored or transmitted, in any form or by any means, without the prior permission in writing of the publishers or in the case of reprographic reproduction in accordance with the terms of licences issued by the Copyright Licensing Agency in the UK, or in accordance with the terms of licences issued by the appropriate Reproduction Rights Organization outside the UK. Enquiries concerning reproduction outside the terms stated here should be sent to the publishers at the UK address printed on this page.

The right of Nicholas J Wald to be identified as author of this work has been asserted by him in accordance with the Copyright, Designs and Patents Act, 1988.

British Library Cataloguing in Publication Data
A catalogue record for this book is available from the British Library

ISBN 1-85315-584-5

Distribution in Europe and Rest of World:
Marston Book Services Ltd
PO Box 269
Abingdon
Oxon OX14 4YN, UK
Tel: +44 (0)1235 465500
Fax: +44 (0)1235 465555

Distribution in the USA and Canada:
Royal Society of Medicine Press Ltd
c/o Jamco Distribution Inc
1401 Lakeway Drive
Lewisville, TX 75057, USA
Tel: +1 800 538 1287
Fax: +1 972 353 1303
E-mail: jamco@majors.com

Distribution in Australia and New Zealand:
Elsevier Australia
30–52 Smidmore Street
Marrickville NSW 2204, Australia
Tel: + 61 2 9517 8999
Fax: +61 2 9517 2249
E-mail: service@elsevier.com.au

Phototypeset by Phoenix Photosetting, Chatham, Kent
Printed and bound in Europe by the Alden Group, Oxford

Contents

'The principal difficulty in your case', remarked Holmes, in his didactic fashion, 'lay in the fact of there being too much evidence. What was vital was overlaid and hidden by what was irrelevant. Of all the facts which were presented to us, we had to pick just those which we deemed to be essential . . .'

Arthur Conan Doyle, *The Naval Treaty*

'I pay the schoolmaster, but 'tis the schoolboys that educate my son.'

Ralph Waldo Emerson, *Journals 1849*

Preface

This book was originally intended as an introduction to epidemiology for medical students, but it has also been found to be of value to doctors and other professionals interested in the subject. It is intended to place epidemiology in the context of medicine as a whole. Increasingly, medical students, doctors and others need to read, assess and interpret an ever-increasing body of medical information. An understanding of the principles of epidemiology is frequently needed when making decisions not only in public health but also in clinical medicine.

From the first edition in 1988, this book has been used at Barts and The London Hospital in connection with the teaching of epidemiology and public health. This edition updates the tables and figures using more recent data from the Office of National Statistics and other sources. Several sections have been revised, in particular those on study design and screening. The use of simple numerical methods (including the meaning of p-values and confidence intervals) has been amended in the light of experience gained in teaching medical students and postgraduates. There is a new section on epidemiological dose–response relations because of the importance of this area in assessing the public health impact of different interventions, such as the quantitative effect of lowering LDL cholesterol in reducing the risk of cardiovascular disease. I have sought to keep *The Epidemiological Approach* brief and simple, offering an insight into the subject and an awareness of its scope and utility, while still being sufficient to be a useful introduction to the subject.

I thank Michael McDowall and Kiran Nanchahal for their help in connection with the first edition of this monograph, and Sir Christopher Booth and Sir Richard Doll for their comments on it. I thank Helen Binns, Patrick Heaton, Carole Parkes, Aubrey Sheiham, David Smith and Karen Wald for their help with the second edition, and Rachel Jordan for her help with the third edition. I thank Frank Speizer, Annie Britten, Leo Kinlen, Jeff Aronson, Jack Canick and Karen Wald for their comments on this edition. I thank Neville Young for his technical assistance and advice. I am most grateful to Dallas Allen for the skill and care with which she produced the manuscript in its many drafts.

I am especially grateful to Malcolm Law and Joan Morris for their help in the preparation of this book and for their many detailed criticisms.

NJW

List of Tables and Figures

Introduction

> **Epidemiology** is the study of the incidence, distribution and determinants of diseases in human populations with a view to identifying their causes and bringing about their prevention.

Epidemiology and clinical medicine are linked, but there is an important distinction between the two. Clinical medicine is concerned with the diagnosis of people who already have a disease and seeks to understand how the disease progresses, what its effects are, and how it can be treated. Epidemiology is concerned with the antecedents of a disease and seeks to identify its causes, thereby making possible its prevention. As such, epidemiology is concerned with populations that necessarily include not only individuals who have the disease in question but also those who do not, thereby permitting the calculation of the rate of occurrence of the disease and hence the study of factors that influence that rate. Clues to what those factors are may be obtained by seeing whether the disease is more common in one place than in another, whether its incidence has changed over time and whether it differs in people with and without certain characteristics.

Epidemiology has also extended its field of interest into areas relevant to clinical medicine. Two are considered further in this book, namely clinical trials and the quantitative interpretation of diagnostic or screening tests, but not others, such as surveillance of the adverse effects of drugs and other medical treatments.

The epidemiologist, like a detective, must usually deduce the factors responsible for causing a disease from naturally occurring circumstances over which he has no control. For example he asks, 'Why is coronary heart disease so much more common in the USA than it is in Japan? Does the risk change when Japanese people migrate to the USA? Is cholesterol, the principal substance in the atheromatous lesions in the coronary arteries, present in different concentrations in the blood of Japanese and Americans? And, within each country, is there an association between serum cholesterol concentration and the risk of coronary heart disease? Is there any evidence that serum cholesterol is not associated with the risk of heart disease?' Only in so far as epidemiologists conduct clinical or prophylactic trials are they experimental scientists. Mostly, however, the epidemiologist's work involves observation and interpretation and especially the study of patterns of morbidity and mortality.

Epidemiology relies on pathology and clinical medicine to define and understand disease, and on statistics to quantify the frequency of disease and the size of the associations with possible causative factors.

A cause of a disease

A cause of a disease increases a person's risk of developing the disease. Risk is a probability that can be applied to an individual from evidence obtained from population studies.

A **cause of a disease** is a factor that is associated with the disease so that if the intensity or prevalence of the factor in a population is changed, the incidence of the disease also changes.

It is obvious that not all associations are causal. For example, alcohol consumption is associated with lung cancer, because cigarette smokers tend to drink more alcohol than non-smokers and smoking is itself associated with lung cancer. The alcohol–lung cancer association is said to be an indirect one, whereas the smoking–lung cancer association is direct and causal. This is supported by the fact that the risk of lung cancer varies according to cigarette consumption in persons with a similar alcohol intake but does *not* vary according to alcohol intake in persons with a similar cigarette consumption. There can be more than one cause of a disease, so that, for example, exposure to arsenic, asbestos or nickel can each independently cause lung cancer. Not everyone exposed to a specific cause of a disease will automatically develop that disease. Most causes of disease are not *necessary* (i.e. one can acquire the disease without the exposure), nor are they *sufficient* (something else is required to result in the disease). For example, not everyone exposed to the tubercle bacillus will develop pulmonary tuberculosis (i.e. it is necessary but not sufficient), and non-smokers can also develop lung cancer (i.e. smoking may be sufficient but it is not necessary). Whether a particular individual develops a disease after such exposures will depend on the interplay of several factors, including the intensity of exposure to other agents, genetic differences, and the play of chance.

An experiment is the most direct way to determine causality, by adding or withholding the suspect factor and observing whether the incidence of the disease changes. Such an experiment, however, often cannot be done in humans when investigating a toxic substance. Removal of the factor may not be possible, the necessary scale of intervention may be too large, or the duration of observation too long, or it may be considered unethical. In such circumstances, causality needs to be inferred from observational studies. This is done in two stages. The first stage is to determine that the data show an association between an exposure and a disease that is unlikely to have arisen by chance (i.e. is likely to be a real association). The second is to assess whether a real association is one of cause and effect.

A real association is most likely to be detected in a study if the magnitude of the association is large, if the study includes a large number of subjects, and by minimising the variation in other factors affecting either the rate of the disease or variation in the measurement of the suspected causal factor, both of which introduce *random error* or 'noise' into the system. Tests of statistical significance help determine whether an association is real.

A real association between a factor and a disease must either be causal or be due to bias or confounding. The exclusion of bias and confounding enables one to infer a causal link. *Bias* arises when an association between a disease and a study factor is due to *systematic* error, which could result from a poorly designed study or from a prejudiced observer. This may occur if an observer who believes that the factor does cause the disease is more likely to diagnose the disease in an individual he knows to have been exposed to the factor; this is *observer* bias and can be avoided by ensuring that the observer who makes the diagnosis of the disease is *blind* to the presence or absence of the factor.

The two types of error – **random error** and **systematic error** – have different consequences. Random error (also called *imprecision*) tends to conceal differences, while systematic error (bias or *inaccuracy*) can introduce a spurious difference (for example, an observer might be more likely to round up blood pressure measurements on a smoker if the observer believes that smoking raises blood pressure). Figure 1 illustrates the difference between precision and accuracy using the analogy of the target patterns of four riflemen.

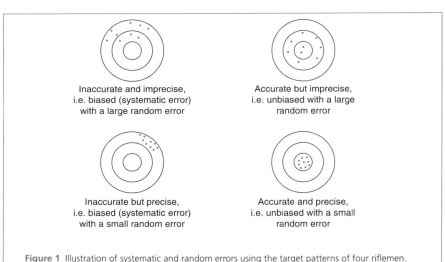

Inaccurate and imprecise, i.e. biased (systematic error) with a large random error

Accurate but imprecise, i.e. unbiased with a large random error

Inaccurate but precise, i.e. biased (systematic error) with a small random error

Accurate and precise, i.e. unbiased with a small random error

Figure 1 Illustration of systematic and random errors using the target patterns of four riflemen.

Random error (or imprecision) can be overcome by increasing sample size in epidemiological studies or clinical trials and by taking several measurements and using the average; systematic error (or bias) cannot be overcome in this way.

Systematic error can only be overcome by good study design that ensures that like is compared with like in every respect other than the factor under study.

In seeking the cause of a disease, error can arise from another source called *confounding*. A confounding factor is one that leads to an indirect association, thereby falsely suggesting one cause of a disease when another is responsible.

> A **confounding factor** is a factor that explains, entirely or in part, an observed association between a study factor and a disease because of its association with both the study factor and the disease.

The observed association between alcohol consumption and lung cancer referred to above suggests that consuming alcohol may cause lung cancer. However, the true explanation for the association is that cigarette smoking is associated with alcohol consumption (drinkers tend to smoke), and smoking causes lung cancer, so the association between alcohol consumption and lung cancer is indirect and not causal. In this example, cigarette smoking is a **confounding** factor and the interrelationships are shown in Figure 2.

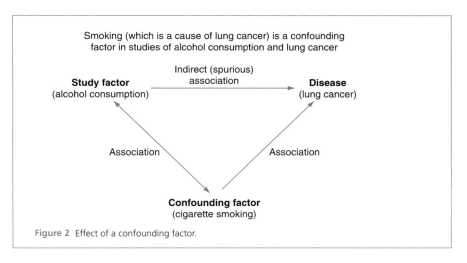

Figure 2 Effect of a confounding factor.

The magnitude of an association provides an indication of whether the association is causal. Strong associations are less likely to have been produced by bias or confounding than small associations. Establishing causality is facilitated by knowledge of the sequence of events involved; it is always a necessary condition of a causal association for the causal factor to precede the effect. This is often clear – for example the association between smoking and lung cancer. At other times it is uncertain, as in an association that was found between low serum retinol and cancer, for which there were two equally plausible explanations: that the low serum retinol preceded the cancer and may therefore have caused it or that the presence of cancer exerted metabolic effects that lowered serum retinol. Only appropriate epidemiological enquiry (a cohort study, see later) was able to determine which explanation was correct, and this (Wald et al, 1986) showed that the low serum retinol preceded the cancer. Once the sequence of events is known it is usually possible to conclude that an association is causal if bias and confounding can be excluded, provided the causal explanation makes biological sense and there is no seriously conflicting evidence. A causal explanation for an association is supported by a dose–response relationship between exposure and the disease, by demonstrating that a reduction in exposure produces a reduction in the incidence of the disease and

---

Table 1

Essential criteria and supporting evidence for inferring causality between an exposure and a disease

---

Essential criteria

1 A real association between the exposure and the disease, that is, an association that is unlikely to be due to chance

2 The exposure precedes the occurrence of the disease

3 The association cannot be reasonably explained by bias (e.g. through systematic measurement error) or through the effect of one or more confounding factors

4 The causal explanation makes biological sense

Supporting evidence

1 The strength of the association; a relative risk* as high as 3 or 4 is less likely to be due to bias than one of 2 or less

2 Consistency in the evidence from several studies that are unlikely to share the same bias

3 Demonstration of a dose–response relationship between the exposure and the disease in studies of individuals

4 The demonstration of reversibility; elimination or reduction in the intensity of exposure is associated with a reduction in the risk of disease

5 The distribution and frequency of the disease in different places and in different groups and over time follows the distribution and intensity of exposure

6 Support from animal or *in vitro* experimental evidence

---

* See page 12 for an explanation of relative risk.

by observing that the variation in the distribution of disease in different places at different times and in different groups of people is related to corresponding variations in the distribution of the causal factor. Table 1 presents in summary form the criteria and evidence for inferring causality between an exposure and a disease.

The definition of the cause of a disease (page 3) stresses the central importance of why a disease occurs rather than how it progresses after it has occurred. The notion of cause is concerned with the origins of disease rather than the mechanisms. The clinician might regard the cause of diabetes as being a relative lack of insulin, while the epidemiologist would want to know what genetic and environmental factors led to this lack. Both views are correct: to treat the acute effects of diabetes, it need only be regarded as a lack of insulin, but to prevent it, it is necessary to understand what factors led to this lack.

Epidemiological enquiry

Epidemiological enquiry involves finding clues to the causes of a disease. Such clues can arise from many sources, for example from clinical observation, from inferences drawn from knowledge of the biology involved, or from a more formal description of the epidemiology of the disease concerned. From such observations and inferences a hypothesis may emerge that a particular disease can be caused by a particular exposure. This can be investigated further in specific epidemiological studies.

Epidemiological studies

Preliminary epidemiological studies involve answering three questions: How does the risk of developing a disease vary over *time*? How does it vary according to *place*? How does it vary with respect to certain characteristics of the *person*, such as age, sex or occupational group?

The risk of developing a disease is determined by estimating the incidence or prevalence of the disease in question, both of which involve counting the number of individuals in a defined population with that disease (the numerator) and dividing by the total population (the denominator) so that disease rates can be determined. The rate at which *new* cases of a disease arise is the *incidence* of the disease.

> The **incidence of a disease** is the number of new cases that occur in a defined population in a specified period of time.
> - The incidence of a particular disease could therefore be expressed as, say, 5 per 1000 persons per year.

The proportion of a population that is *already affected* by a particular disease at a particular time is the *prevalence* of the disease.

> The **prevalence of a disease** is the number of cases of a disease present in a defined population at a given point in time.
> - The prevelance of a particular disease could therefore be expressed as, say, 5 per 1000 persons.

The prevalence of a disease changes according to the product of its incidence and duration. The duration of a disease is shortened either if it kills the patient or if it remits completely. A condition with a high incidence and a low prevalence could therefore be either a common disease with a high fatality rate (e.g. lung cancer) or a common disease with a high remission rate (e.g. measles). A disease with a low incidence and a high prevalence will be a chronic disease with a low fatality rate and a low remission rate (e.g. rheumatoid arthritis).

The prevalence and incidence of a disease are usually strongly dependent on age. For example, the incidences of coronary heart disease and most cancers are relatively high in the elderly and low in the young. When comparing incidence or prevalence across different communities, say, India and Britain, it can be misleading to compare the overall rates directly since one population may have a large number of elderly people while the other may have few. One approach to the problem is to make separate comparisons for each five- or ten-year age group, although such comparisons are unwieldy since they do not yield a single summary figure. This can be obtained by 'age standardisation' in which the death rates are calculated that would be expected to occur if the study population had the same age structure as the standard population. There are two methods – direct and indirect, depending on whether the age-specific death rates are taken from the study population (direct standardisation) or from the standard population (indirect standardisation). In *direct* standardisation, one first multiplies the age- and sex-specific death rates in the population under study by the corresponding numbers of individuals in the standard population. This yields the number of deaths that would have been expected in the corresponding age/sex groups in the standard population if that population had experienced the same death rates as the study population. These deaths are then summed and the total number of deaths is divided by the number of people in the standard population. The resulting death rate is thus directly standardised for age and sex and can be compared with the rate from another population standardised in the same way.

In *indirect* standardisation, one starts with the age- and sex-specific death rates in a standard population – not those in the study population. These rates are then multiplied by the corresponding numbers of individuals in each age/sex group in the study population. This yields the number of observed deaths that would have been expected in the corresponding age/sex groups in the study population if that population had experienced the same death rates as the standard population. The total number of deaths in the study population is then divided by the sum of all these expected deaths and multiplied by 100. The resulting rate is the standardised mortality ratio (SMR). If it is over 100, the mortality rate is higher than in the standard population; for example, an SMR of 120 indicates a death rate 20% higher than the standard population. If it is under 100, the mortality rate is lower than in the standard population. The SMR times the death rate in the standard population is the rate indirectly standardised for age and sex.

Although people may think that a direct estimate is better than an indirect one, in practice indirect standardisation is better and more widely used. This is because the standard population is almost always much larger than the study population, so that the age- and sex-specific death rates will be more reliable than those based on the study population.

Life expectancy is another important summary measure for comparing death rates within and between countries over time (see Figure 18). It is calculated by considering a hypothetical group of, say, 1000 individuals at a given age and applying to the group the age-specific death rates of the population for each year of age until the whole group is estimated to have died. Expectation of life is calculated as the total number of person-years of life lived by the group divided by the number in the group, i.e. the average number of years an individual is expected on average to live. The calculation assumes that the current death rates will remain unchanged for the lifetime of the group, which, of course, they will not; however, expectation of life is a useful single index of *current* death rates.

A description of the differences in the epidemiological characteristics of a disease over time, from place to place, and among different groups of people within a place can be useful, because, as well as the burden of disease (in both economic and health terms), it can suggest clues to the causes of the disease. Such studies are sometimes called descriptive epidemiological studies because they study diseases and suspect exposures in groups as a whole. The study of immigrants is especially helpful. For example, the Japanese have a high incidence of stomach cancer but this falls substantially in Japanese migrants who move to the USA, where the incidence rates in the Japanese approximate to those of indigenous Americans within one or two generations. The incidence of colon cancer is low in Japan but in Japanese immigrants it increases towards the level in indigenous Americans. There must be an agent that causes stomach cancer to which the Japanese are more heavily exposed than the Americans. Similarly there must be an agent that causes colon cancer to which the Americans are more heavily exposed than the Japanese.

Once a hypothesis has been produced postulating that a particular disease is caused by a particular exposure, the epidemiological characteristics of the exposure can be described in much the same way as the epidemiology of the disease to see if the two are correlated with respect to time and place, and to see if the two tend to occur together in certain groups of people within the same community. Such studies can test a hypothesis as well as generating aetiological clues.

Measures of risk used in epidemiological studies

Once preliminary epidemiological studies point to a possible association between an exposure and a disease, the possibility can be explored further by performing additional studies specially designed to investigate directly the risk of a disease in relation to a given exposure. It is simplest to consider first the measures of risk used and then the usual study designs employed.

Incidence rates (or mortality rates) in two groups of people – say, among smokers and non-smokers – can be compared in two ways. One rate can be divided by the

> The **relative risk of a disease** in relation to a particular exposure is the incidence of a disease among exposed persons divided by the incidence among unexposed persons.

> The **absolute excess risk of a disease** in relation to a particular exposure is the incidence of the disease among exposed persons minus the incidence among non-exposed persons.

other to give the ratio of the rates to derive the relative risk, or alternatively one can be subtracted from the other to determine the absolute difference between the rates.

The relative risk gives the strength of an association, which can help in determining if the association is causal. If causal, the absolute excess risk is a direct measure of how much disease the exposure causes in a particular population, indicating the effect of removing the exposure from the population; it is therefore of public health value. Because the absolute excess risk depends on the underlying risk of the disease in the unexposed members of a particular population, it may not apply to other populations.

Table 2 shows the relative risk and absolute excess risk for mortality from lung cancer,

Table 2

Relative and absolute risks of death from selected causes associated with cigarette smoking in British male physicians

Cause of death	Age-standardised annual death rate per 100 000		Relative risk	Absolute excess risk (death rate per 100 000 per yr)
	Non-smokers	Current smokers		
Lung cancer	14	209	$\frac{209}{14}$ = 14.9	209–14 = 195
Chronic obstructive lung disease	10	127	$\frac{127}{10}$ = 12.7	127–10 = 117
Ischaemic heart disease	542	892	$\frac{892}{542}$ = 1.6	892–542 = 350
All causes	1706	3038	$\frac{3038}{1706}$ = 1.8	3038–1706 = 1332

Source: Doll R, Peto R, Wheatley K et al. Mortality in relation to smoking: 40 years' observations on male British doctors. *BMJ* 1994; **309**: 901–11.

chronic bronchitis, and cardiovascular disease in cigarette smokers and non-smokers.

Smoking is an important cause of lung cancer and of chronic obstructive lung disease, as evidenced by their high relative risks (14.9 and 12.7 respectively in current smokers). However, because of the relative rarity of the two diseases in non-smokers, smoking causes fewer deaths from these diseases (195 and 117 deaths per 100 000 per year respectively among smokers) than deaths from ischaemic heart disease (350 deaths per 100 000 per year), even though the relative risk of ischaemic heart disease in smokers is only 1.6. Even though the mortality of a common disease is increased only about two times, the final number of deaths is greater than a rare disease being increased by as much as 15 times.

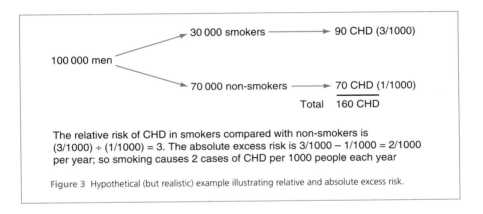

The relative risk of CHD in smokers compared with non-smokers is (3/1000) ÷ (1/1000) = 3. The absolute excess risk is 3/1000 − 1/1000 = 2/1000 per year; so smoking causes 2 cases of CHD per 1000 people each year

Figure 3 Hypothetical (but realistic) example illustrating relative and absolute excess risk.

Figure 3 presents a simple hypothetical (but realistic) example to illustrate relative risk and absolute excess risk, and to show how the attributable proportion is calculated. In a population of 100 000 men aged 45–54 years, 30% are smokers, and the risk of dying from coronary heart disease (CHD) is 3 per 1000 per year among smokers and 1 per 1000 per year among non-smokers. The relative risk in this example is higher than that shown in Table 2 (1.6) because it relates to younger men, among whom the relative risk due to smoking is greater.

If no one smoked, there would be 100 deaths (100 000 × 1/1000) instead of 160, i.e. 60 out of the 160 observed deaths are due to smoking. The proportion of deaths attributable to smoking in this population is therefore 60/160 or 38%. To estimate the attributable proportion, one need not know the absolute death rates in smokers and non-smokers, but simply the relative risk (RR) and the prevalence of the exposure (P) (Figure 4). If more of the population smoked, the attributable proportion would be higher; this measure therefore varies from one population to another, depending on the prevalence and extent of exposure.

> The **attributable proportion** is the proportion of cases of a disease that can be attributed to an exposure.

$$\text{Attributable proportion} = \frac{P(RR-1)}{P(RR-1)+1}$$

$$\text{which, in our example} = \frac{0.3(3-1)}{0.3(3-1)+1} = \frac{0.6}{1.6} = 38\%$$

(P = prevalence of exposure, RR = relative risk)

Figure 4 Attributable proportion.

Dose–response relationships

A single relative risk estimate applies to a categorical exposure such as smoking, irrespective of the amount smoked. If the exposure can be considered quantitatively, such as the number of cigarettes smoked per day, there are several relative risk estimates, each corresponding to a different smoking group (say 1–5, 6–9, 10–14, etc cigarettes per day) and if the relative risk increases with cigarette consumption then a dose–response effect is present. For risk factors that are continuous variables (e.g. cholesterol and heart disease, blood pressure and stroke, or bone density and hip fracture), we need to specify a change in risk for a specified change in the exposure or level of the risk factor. This is done using a *regression analysis* in which the incidence of disease in increasing categories of the risk factor is plotted on a graph and the '*best fit line*' between the two is estimated. Such an analysis makes it possible to quantify the relationship between a risk factor and the risk of a disease caused by the risk factor. This enables one to judge the extent to which a change in the risk factor reduces the risk of the disease.

There are three general types of dose–response relationships, depending on whether a linear dose–response relationship is achieved by plotting the risk factor and/or the incidence of disease on an (absolute) arithmetic or a (proportional) logarithmic scale. For example, in Figure 5, the relative risk of dying from a stroke is plotted against diastolic blood pressure on (a) two arithmetic scales, (b) a logarithmic scale and an arithmetic one and (c) two logarithmic scales. Visually, graph (b) is the straightest line. This is of considerable importance. It means that the dose–response relationship can be interpreted as a constant proportional change in the risk of stroke death for a specified absolute change in diastolic blood pressure. For example, a change of 8 mmHg doubles the risk of a stroke **regardless**

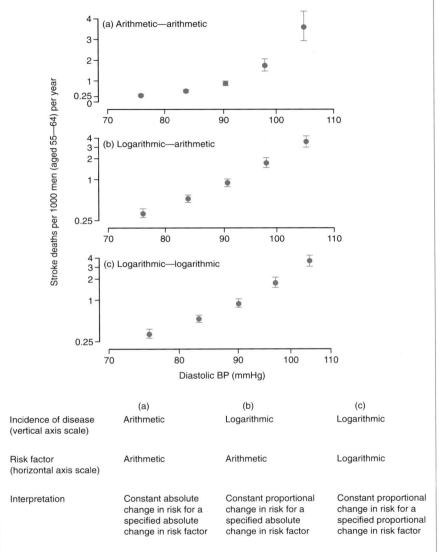

Figure 5 Arithmetic and logarithmic (proportional) scales in determining dose–response relationships. *Source*: Law MR, Wald NJ. Risk factor thresholds: their existence under scrutiny. *BMJ* 2003; **324:** 1570–6.

of the initial blood pressure. In the association between risk and a continuously distributed variable, it is helpful to be able to derive a straight line relationship, because the slope of a straight line is generalisable from one population to another and is the same whatever the starting level of the risk factor. To define a straight line relationship, it is necessary to specify the intercept and the slope of the line, called a *regression line*. Usually the intercept has no practical application, but the slope is important and generalisable. The relation that best yields a straight line is the one of choice.

Study design

Epidemiological studies based on data relating to individuals are either prospective or retrospective. They are observational studies using data relating to individuals in a group rather than to the groups as a whole (descriptive epidemiological studies).

In a *cohort* (or *prospective*) study, we take a group of individuals and categorise each according to whether they are exposed to the factor under investigation, which may for example be smoking, a certain food, an infection or a blood level. We then follow these individuals for a period of time, say ten or more years, and record those who develop the disease of interest. Determining which individuals develop the disease is generally done by linkage to death certification data or cancer registries; identifying non-fatal disease events other than cancer may be difficult unless contact is maintained with the study participants. A simple 2×2 table of the number of individuals involved can be constructed to present the results as in Table 3.

Table 3

Presentation of results from a cohort (or a case–control) study

	Disease	No disease	Total
Exposed	a	b	$a+b$
Not exposed	c	d	$c+d$
Total	$a+c$	$b+d$	n

There are thus $a+c$ cases of disease in total, so the incidence is $(a+c)/n$ per ten years if everyone was followed up for ten years.

The measures of risk are then calculated as in the example in Figure 3. Using the notation in Table 3, the rates of disease in exposed subjects, $a/(a+b)$, and in unexposed subjects, $c/(c+d)$, are determined; the first rate divided by the second is the *relative risk*, $a/(a+b) \div c/(c+d)$, which indicates the number of times exposed subjects are more likely to develop the disease than unexposed subjects. A value for $a/(a+b) \div c/(c+d)$ that is statistically significantly greater than, or less than, 1 is evidence of an association. The second rate subtracted from the first is the *absolute excess risk*, $a/(a+b) - c/(c+d)$.

Table 4 gives a hypothetical but realistic example of data from a cohort study of smoking and lung cancer.

The main *advantages* of **cohort** studies are:

  (i) the knowledge that the exposure preceded the occurrence of the disease;
 (ii) the ability to obtain a direct estimate of the incidence of the disease in the exposed and the unexposed groups (this allows not only the relative risk to be estimated directly but also the absolute excess risk);
(iii) the ability to detect other diseases associated with the exposure;
 (iv) the ability to study rare exposures (e.g. special occupational groups).

Their main *disadvantages* when studying chronic disorders, such as cardiovascular disease and cancer, are:

  (i) their long duration (often many years);
 (ii) their large size (thousands of individuals); and therefore
(iii) their financial cost – for a rare disease, few cases may develop, even in a large study of this type.

Table 4

Hypothetical (but realistic) example of a cohort study of smoking and lung cancer

Initial population of 100 000	Ten-year follow-up of new cases of lung cancer	
	Number	**Rate**
30 000 smokers	225	225/30 000 = 75/10 000
70 000 non-smokers	35	35/70 000 = 5/10 000

Relative risk, $r = \dfrac{75/10\ 000}{5/10\ 000} = 15$, i.e. smokers are 15 times more likely to get lung cancer than non-smokers

Absolute excess risk, $e = 75/1000 - 5/10\ 000 = 70/10\ 000/10$ years
$= 7/10\ 000/\text{year}$

Note that the estimate of relative risk, 15, is similar to that for lung cancer in Table 2, but the absolute excess risk is lower (7 compared with 19.5 per 10 000 per year). The most likely explanation would be that the study population here is younger, so the incidence is lower

In a *case–control* (or *retrospective*) *study*, we take a sample of individuals who have the disease (cases) and another sample who do not (controls). The prevalence of the past (hence retrospective) exposure to the factor under study in those with the disease and in those without it is determined, usually by a questionnaire.

Table 5

Approximation permitting the calculation of relative risk from a case–control study

(1) For a cohort study, using the terms shown in Table 3, the relative risk,

$$RR = a/(a+b) \div c/(c+d)$$

If the disease is rare then a is much smaller than b, and c is much smaller than d, so

(i) $a+b$ is approximately equal to b, and $a/(a+b)$ is approximately equal to a/b;

(ii) $c+d$ is approximately equal to d, and $c/(c+d)$ is approximately equal to c/d.

Therefore, the relative risk, RR, is approximately equal to $a/b \div c/d = ad/bc$. This ratio ($a/b \div c/d$) is called the **odds ratio** (or **relative odds**). It compares the number in mutually exclusive categories ($a/b \div c/d$), whereas the relative risk [$a/(a+b) \div c/(c+d)$] does not, since the numerator is part of the denominator (a is in both). However, the relative odds is a good estimate of the relative risk if the disease is rare.

(2) Similarly, for a case–control study, let s_1 and s_2 be the unknown fractions of individuals with and without the disease sampled from the underlying population to yield, respectively, the number of cases and the number of controls in the study.

Then the odds ratio (**the estimate of the relative risk**),

$$
\begin{aligned}
OR &= as_1/bs_2 \div cs_1/ds_2 \\
&= as_1/bs_2 \times ds_2/cs_1 \\
&= ad/bc, \text{ since } s_1 \text{ and } s_2 \text{ cancel}
\end{aligned}
$$

i.e. the ratio of the cross-products of the 2×2 table.

The unknown sampling fractions s_1 and s_2 have conveniently cancelled out, leaving the odds ratio OR as a close approximation to the true relative risk as shown in (1) above, if the disease is rare.

In a case–control study, we cannot estimate the incidence of the disease, because the proportion of diseased subjects in the population is unknown. However, if the disease being studied is rare, the relative risk can be derived, since a simple approximation solves the problem (Table 5). Table 6 shows an example.

The results in Table 6 are in certain respects remarkable. In 1950, the prevalence of current and ex-smokers was extremely high: 95% in the study concerned (1269/1298). Had everyone been smokers, we may never have known that smoking was a cause of lung cancer. Fortunately, there were 5% of people who had never smoked, and these provided the necessary comparison group. It is worth reflecting that in epidemiology, if a population is completely unexposed to an agent, or if everyone is exposed to that agent, then it is impossible to determine whether that agent may be a cause of a disease. It is the variation that allows us to identify possible causes.

Table 6

Case–control study of lung cancer and cigarette smoking among men

Smoking habits	Cases (lung cancer)	Controls (no lung cancer)	Total
Cigarette smokers	647	622	1269
Non-smokers	2	27	29
Total	649	649	1298

Odds ratio (estimate of relative risk), OR $= \dfrac{647 \times 27}{622 \times 2} = 14$

Source: Doll R, Hill AB. Smoking and carcinoma of the lung. *BMJ* 1950; **ii**: 739–48.

The main *advantages* of **case–control** studies are that they:

(i) are quick;

(ii) require relatively small numbers;

(iii) are hence reasonably economical;

(iv) are sometimes the only feasible way to conduct an observational epidemiological study of a rare disease.

Their main *disadvantages* are:

(i) the difficulty, sometimes, of determining whether the exposure preceded the inception of the disease;

(ii) *recall bias*; for example, sick people may be more likely to recall a past exposure than healthy controls;

(iii) the possibility of *selection bias*, in which the recruitment of cases and controls is influenced by whether or not they have been exposed;

(iv) the inability to obtain a direct estimate of incidence, and hence to estimate excess risk, in exposed and unexposed groups.

There are two important variants of cohort studies: (i) a *historical cohort study* and (ii) a design that (perhaps confusingly) is called a *nested case–control study*. A historical cohort study identifies a large group of individuals who are documented as having an exposure a long time ago, say 50 years in the past. These are followed up usually to determine whether the subjects have died and, if so, the cause of death. Since most of the deaths will have already occurred, there is no need to wait many years as in a conventional cohort study. This therefore has the merits of a cohort study and much of the advantage of being able to obtain a quick result associated with case–control studies. The second variant, the nested case–control study, is performed within a large cohort study when it would be difficult or expensive to carry out measurements on all the individuals in the study. For example, if blood samples were collected from all the subjects at enrolment and stored in freezers, then, after a period of follow-up, the blood test may be performed on the samples from those individuals who developed the disease of interest (cases) together with only a sample of the unaffected individuals (controls), matched to the cases. The following illustrates the nested case–control design. In a cohort study of 20 000 persons after 20 years follow-up, 600 had died of heart disease. If we want to determine whether those with antibodies to certain infectious agents were more likely to have died of heart disease, it would not be necessary to test all 20 000 blood samples for the antibodies, but only the samples from the 600 who died of heart disease and a control group of, say, 600 selected from the 19 400 who did not die of heart disease. The 600 controls would be selected to match the cases by age, sex and possibly other criteria. Such a nested case–control study is, from an epidemiological perspective, a cohort study, but with some of the economies of a standard case–control study.

Intervention studies

Intervention studies resemble cohort studies in that subjects are followed up to determine their outcome. They differ in that some action or intervention is performed rather than merely observing what takes place naturally. Intervention studies are experiments in which a regimen is administered to an experimental group and the observed outcome is compared with a control group that is not given the regimen. If there is a difference in outcome between the two groups and the difference is considered unlikely to have arisen by chance and unlikely to be due to bias, cause and effect can be inferred.

In general, three types of control groups can be used:

(i) *historical controls*, patients with the same disorder seen in the past before the use of the new intervention;
(ii) *geographical controls*, patients with the same disorder seen at another hospital or clinic where the new intervention is not provided;
(iii) *randomised controls*.

Two types of randomised controls can be used: (a) a 'parallel group', comprising patients allocated at random to a treated or a control group, and (b) a 'crossover group', comprising patients who act as their own controls; for example, a blood pressure-lowering drug could be used for three months and a placebo for three months and the blood pressure change over the two periods compared. The sequence of administering the new drug or the placebo is determined at random. Figure 6 illustrates the two types of randomised group trials.

Randomisation

Randomised trials are conducted to avoid bias by ensuring that like is compared with like and the regimen is the *only* systematic difference between the study and

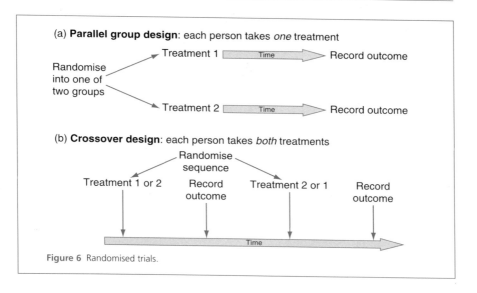

Figure 6 Randomised trials.

control groups. In *parallel group* trials, small chance differences between the groups in other factors that influence outcome will vary randomly in different directions and, if the trial is big enough, will balance each other on average. The main advantage of crossover trials is that by limiting the comparison of interest to within-person differences, the study has greater statistical power. It avoids the 'noise' or extra random variation that arises from between-person differences. It is therefore easier to determine a genuine drug effect against the background random variation in the population. Crossover designs are not always possible; for example, if there is a long carry-over effect or if the endpoint of interest is a single critical event, such as cancer recurrence or death. The use of historical and geographical controls is usually unsatisfactory because there is no way of ensuring that like is being compared with like, so bias can result. The introduction of a new treatment can itself alter the selection of patients referred for the treatment; for example, patients with early disease may start coming from other centres to receive the new treatment. Past patients may have been referred to hospitals at a different stage of the disease, and this alone will influence their survival or remission rate. They may also have received different treatments apart from the new one under study, and this may influence their outcomes. Similar biases affect the use of geographical controls.

A randomised study (or trial) is not one conducted on a random sample of patients; the patients are often a special subset, for example those with a particular complication in a particular age group or those thought likely to comply with the treatment. It is the allocation to receive or not receive the new regimen that is conducted at random, not the selection of the whole group of patients for the study.

Randomisation avoids *selection bias*, that is bias that arises when patients who receive the new treatment have a systematically better or worse prognosis than the controls. Bias that arises when patients know that they are receiving a particular regimen – for example because of a *placebo* effect or because taking the treatment may alter other aspects of behaviour (e.g. exercise, use of vitamins or other medication) that itself affect prognosis – can be avoided by using a *single-blind* design, in which the patients do not know the treatment allocation. With a *double-blind* design, neither the observers nor the patients know the treatment allocation. This ensures that (i) the use of other potential treatments, (ii) the assessment of outcome and (iii) the decision to withdraw a patient who is, say, not doing well in the study cannot be influenced by a clinician's or patient's knowledge of the treatment being used. A double-blind trial is not always feasible, but often at least the assessment of the outcome can be done by observers who are unaware of the allocation to treatment. The main statistical analysis of randomised trials should be a comparison of the outcomes in *all* the subjects who are randomised into the study. Patients who do not take the treatment (so-called non-compliers) are not excluded from the analysis. This *intention-to-treat* analysis, rather than one that compares outcomes only in patients who actually complete the treatment (*on-treatment analysis*), is the only way of being sure that bias is avoided. Bias could easily be introduced in an on-treatment analysis because, for example, the more symptomatic patients with a poorer prognosis may be less likely to adhere to one treatment than the other, particularly if it has adverse effects that exacerbate the symptoms from the disease itself, such as nausea. Omitting the non-compliers from the analysis can make the outcome in the rest of the treated group appear better, or worse, than that in the controls, even if the treatment was in fact useless. Poor compliance on an intention-to-treat analysis will reduce the ability of the trial to detect a treatment effect if one does exist (i.e. a trial with poor compliance will have little statistical power and may yield inconclusive results) but it will avoid selection bias. However, the estimate of the treatment effect will be diluted.

An intention-to-treat analysis also addresses the pragmatic question 'Did the new treatment work in practice?' That is, 'How much benefit, if any, is there among those for whom the new treatment was presented?' rather than 'How much benefit, if any is there among those who take it?' A pharmacologically effective treatment that is rejected because it is so disagreeable is of little value, although knowledge that it may be effective is important because it will keep the door open in the search for other similar drugs that may be more acceptable and just as effective.

A randomised trial can be used to investigate the value of more than one treatment, by randomising patients into a control group and several experimental groups. This approach will involve the recruitment of more patients into the trial. A way of avoiding this increased cost is to use a *factorial design*. If two new drugs are being evaluated, this involves randomising the population into four groups: one to receive neither drug, two to receive one drug only and one to receive both. The main advantage is that each treatment is given to half the available patients, rather than to one-third, increasing statistical power so that two drugs can be assessed using the same number of patients needed to assess one drug. If each drug exerted opposite effects or if they interfered with each other in such a way as to reduce the effect of any one alone, this would be a weak design, but it is only by using such a design that these and other *treatment interactions* can be studied. Large numbers of patients are, however, usually needed to do this reliably.

An example of a factorial design is the ISIS-2 study (ISIS, 1988). Here, 17 187 patients who entered 417 hospitals up to 24 hours after the onset of a suspected acute myocardial infarction were randomised between: (i) streptokinase, a 1-hour intravenous infusion of 1.5 MU; (ii) aspirin, 1 month of 160 mg/day, enteric-coated; (iii) both treatments; or (iv) neither (double placebo control). Table 7 shows the incidence of 5-week vascular mortality (IHD and stroke) following these regimens.

Table 7

Five-week vascular mortality in 17 187 treated patients with suspected myocardial infarction (deaths/no. of patients)

| | | Streptokinase | | |
		Yes	No	Total
Aspirin	**Yes**	$\dfrac{343}{4292}$	$\dfrac{461}{4295}$	$\dfrac{804}{8587}$
	No	$\dfrac{448}{4300}$	$\dfrac{568}{4300}$	$\dfrac{1016}{8600}$
Total		$\dfrac{791}{8592}$	$\dfrac{1029}{8595}$	$\dfrac{1820}{17\ 187}$

Comparison of aspirin vs no aspirin

Comparison of streptokinase vs no streptokinase

Source: ISIS. Randomised trial of intravenous streptokinase, oral aspirin, both, or neither among 17 187 cases of suspected acute myocardial infarction: ISIS-2. *Lancet* 1988; **ii:** 349–59.

The results can be summarised in the following way:

Relative risk reduction*

1. Effect of streptokinase alone (S)

$$S \text{ vs no } S = \frac{791}{8592} \text{ (9.2%)} \qquad \text{vs} \qquad \frac{1029}{8595} \text{ (12.0%)} \quad 23\% \left[\frac{12.0-9.2}{12.0\%} \right]$$

2. Effect of aspirin alone (A)

$$A \text{ vs no } A = \frac{804}{8587} \text{ (9.4%)} \qquad \text{vs} \qquad \frac{1016}{8600} \text{ (11.8%)} \quad 20\% \left[\frac{11.8-9.4}{11.8\%} \right]$$

3. Effect of streptokinase and aspirin combined (S+A)

$$S+A \text{ vs no } S \text{ or } A \frac{343}{4292} \text{ (8.0%)} \qquad \text{vs} \qquad \frac{568}{4300} \text{ (13.2%)} \quad 39\% \left[\frac{13.2-8.0}{13.2\%} \right]$$

(*odds compare mutually exclusive groups, e.g. in the S category 791/(8592−791) instead of 791/8592)

Conclusion: Streptokinase alone and aspirin alone significantly reduce vascular mortality; both together are better than each alone, and the effect of each is independent of the other.

Ethical issues

In observational studies in which data are obtained from existing medical records, the ethical issue of concern is maintaining the confidentiality of the records. Much useful information of public benefit can be obtained in this way without harm, and it is important not to discourage such research. Discouragement can unwittingly arise from an insistence that access to records be prohibited unless the subjects themselves give explicit consent or each enquiry requires special permission before access is granted. If the data are obtained by interviewing subjects then the questions asked and the manner of working should be designed in such a way as to avoid causing anxiety. Observational studies represent one of the most harmless and unintrusive forms of medical enquiry. In an intervention study, there is the further ethical concern that patients must not be harmed, either by too high an incidence of serious adverse effects of the new treatment or by withholding it, if it were of benefit. Investigators are naturally enthusiastic about the possible benefits of a new 'treatment' with which they have been associated and they are often understandably unwilling to carry out a controlled experiment to test its effects. It is important, however, to be objective, since many supposedly beneficial treatments have been introduced, but have subsequently been found to be of little or no value, and sometimes even to be harmful, the initial impression of benefit having been due to bias or chance. Assessing the level of certainty over the benefits and hazards of a new intervention requires dispassionate judgement. A practical indication that such uncertainty exists is often the varying practice of clinicians, some avoiding a new treatment on account of scepticism of its value and possibly even fear of its risks but others offering it because of their conviction that it is effective. In such circumstances, a formal randomised trial is a practical and ethical way of settling diversity in clinical practice so that the uncertainty can be resolved. New medical procedures are best evaluated early, before they become uncritically universally accepted.

There is often a perception that in clinical medicine there is a tension between good research and sound ethics and clinical practice. In reality, the two work in harmony. If there is certainty about the value of a treatment, it is bad research to investigate it and unethical to deny some people the benefits of that treatment. However, if there is uncertainty over the value of a treatment, it is ethical to be honest and forthcoming about the uncertainty and good research to conduct a clinical trial to find out. If an early result emerges, for example showing that a treatment under study is clearly more effective than a placebo (or an alternative treatment used), the trial can be stopped early. For this reason, it is usual for an independent data monitoring committee to review the conduct of the trial and to advise on early stopping.

Confidence intervals and *p*-values

Confidence intervals indicate the range of values that is likely to include the true value (Box 1). For example, if we wanted to know what proportion of the population were smokers and we asked a sample of 100 people from the population whether they smoke, and 30 say they did, then we can calculate that the 95% confidence interval is 21–39. This means that we can be 95% certain that the mean prevalence of smoking (i.e. the prevalence in the entire population) is 30% and the

---

Box 1

95% confidence interval

What is meant by the 95% confidence interval?

The 95% confidence interval is the range of values within which one can be 95% certain that the true value occurs

What is meant by '95% certain'?

If the same study were repeated 100 times in 95 of these studies, the confidence intervals would include the true value, but in 5 it would not

Could this be shown to be correct?

Yes. If you carried out the study on the whole population, you would obtain the true value, and with this you could check that the above was correct

true prevalence lies within the interval 21–39%. By '95% certain' we mean that if we repeated the same survey 100 times, the true result would fall outside the range of the confidence interval five times. If we had sampled only 10 people and 3 said they smoked, our point estimate would still be 30% but it would be subject to greater uncertainty – the 95% confidence interval would be 2–58%; if 1000 were sampled and 300 said they smoked, the confidence interval would be tight (27–33%) and the estimate more precise; larger numbers reduce random error.

Confidence intervals tell us nothing about bias (systematic error). For example, if smokers in general tend to deny smoking when they in fact do smoke, this would yield an inaccurate estimate of the prevalence of smoking that would not be suggested by the confidence interval, or corrected by larger numbers. Only good study design with, if necessary, appropriate validation can avoid this kind of systematic error.

In a clinical trial comparing the reduction in blood pressure produced by two drugs, the confidence interval could be applied to the reduction achieved by each drug, but it is more useful to apply it to the *difference* in effect between the two. If one drug, on average, lowered blood pressure by 10 mmHg more than the other, and the 95% confidence interval was narrow (e.g. 8–12 mmHg), we could be reasonably sure of the magnitude of the difference in effects between the two drugs. With a wider confidence interval (e.g. 1–19 mmHg) we would be less sure.

In a negative trial, tight confidence intervals (e.g. –2 to +2 mmHg) exclude the likelihood that a big difference has been missed. Wider confidence intervals spanning 0 (e.g. –10 to +10 mmHg) indicate that the result of the trial is inconclusive: a big difference may have been missed or there could be no difference. It is for this reason that when clinical trials are properly planned, a sufficiently large number of patients is needed to give sufficient statistical power to detect or exclude a clinically important effect.

Confidence intervals can also be applied to relative risk estimates from observational studies and clinical trials. A relative risk of 1.0 indicates no difference, so a relative risk estimate that has a 95% confidence interval that includes 1.0 would not be statistically significant.

Probability (p) values indicate the probability that an observed effect, or one more extreme, would be expected to have arisen by chance alone. So, for example, a difference between two treatments with a p-value below 0.05 means that if there were, in reality, no underlying difference then one would observe a difference as extreme or more extreme than the observed one less than 5 times in 100 similar studies or trials. Statistically, this is said to be a test of the null hypothesis rejected at the $p < 0.05$ level. A p-value is analogous to a false-positive rate as used in screening terminology (see Appendix III).

Confidence intervals are related to p-values. If the 95% confidence interval includes a no-difference result (a relative risk of 1.0 or a difference of 0.0), the observed result is not statistically significant.

Different confidence intervals correspond to different levels of statistical significance (Box 2).

Box 2

Relation between confidence intervals and levels of statistical significance

Confidence intervals excluding no difference	Level of equivalent statistical significance (*p*-value)
95%	0.05
99%	0.01
99.9%	0.001

It is important to recognise that a result that is statistically significant need not be clinically important; it is simply a result that is unlikely to have occurred by chance. Also, *p*-values, like confidence intervals, indicate the likely effect of chance and say nothing about the effect of bias.

Confidence intervals are generally more useful than *p*-values, as they provide more information: they not only indicate whether the result may have been a fluke but also indicate the range of values that is likely to include the true value, that is, they indicate the precision of the estimate.

Prevention

Epidemiology, with its emphasis on identifying the antecedents of disease, offers opportunities for disease prevention. Different measures can be applied at different stages in the natural history of a disease. Primary prevention aims to remove the cause – for example, in the case of lung cancer by the avoidance of smoking, or the prevention of an infectious disease by increasing host resistance, either by general measures (e.g. improving nutrition) or by specific measures (e.g. immunisation). Secondary prevention is the prevention of overt (clinical) cases of a disorder through screening followed by appropriate intervention, as in breast cancer screening by mammography. The treatment of clinical disease, while not normally regarded as prevention, is sometimes referred to as tertiary prevention, in recognition of the fact that effective treatment can prevent disability and pain resulting from the disease.

Primary prevention

The prevention of disease through general social and economic changes that improve nutrition, increase living standards, lead to smaller families and reduce overcrowding is extremely important, even if the precise causal factors involved are difficult to identify. Very poor countries can have extremely low expectations of life, for example under 40 years of age in Zambia (Figure 7); countries with a gross national product (GNP) greater than about $10 000 per person tend to have expectations of life that often have little relationship to GNP, or to health care expenditure.

Past improvements in life expectancy in developed countries were due largely to general measures such as improvements in nutrition and living standards that led to the primary prevention of common infectious diseases. Thus mortality from infectious diseases decreased greatly after the availability of immunisation or antibiotics. Some infectious diseases have increased in frequency, particularly sexually transmitted diseases such as nongonococcal urethritis and more recently acquired immune deficiency syndrome (AIDS). With the notable exception of AIDS, the major challenge today in the industrialised countries of the world is the prevention of non-infectious diseases by specific risk factor modification, using drugs and in changing cultural and personal patterns of behaviour such as in the consumption of specific dietary components (e.g. lower fat and salt intake), increasing levels of physical activity, avoidance of obesity, the prudent consumption of alcohol and the avoidance of tobacco. The adoption throughout Western countries of a diet that would reduce serum cholesterol concentration by 10% would be expected to reduce coronary heart disease mortality by about 27% at age 60 (Law et al, 1994). Since this is the leading cause of death in such countries, such a reduction would be enormous in terms of the number of deaths prevented – approximately equivalent to the complete eradication of lung cancer in men and breast cancer in women. Also important, particularly among young adults, are deaths and injury from accidents, especially road traffic accidents. Society can influence health in various ways, for example by legislation on driving and alcohol consumption, and on air, soil and water pollution, by encouraging the alteration of the composition and quality of food (for example food fortification with folic acid to prevent neural tube defects and cardiovascular disease), through financial incentives (increasing the duty on cigarettes), and by applying engineering principles to build safety into the design of motor vehicles, equipment, buildings and highways.

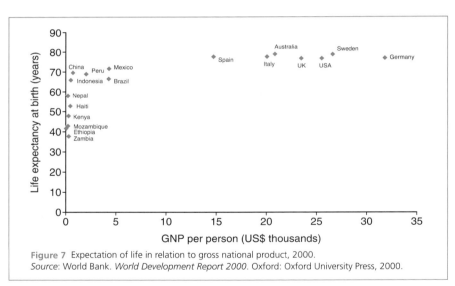

Figure 7 Expectation of life in relation to gross national product, 2000.
Source: World Bank. *World Development Report 2000*. Oxford: Oxford University Press, 2000.

Screening

Screening is the systematic application of a test or enquiry, to identify individuals at sufficient risk of a specific disorder to benefit from further investigation or direct preventive action, among persons who have not sought medical attention on account of symptoms of that disorder.

Screening (usually a form of secondary prevention) represents a radical departure from traditional medicine, since it is usually concerned with the detection of disorders at an asymptomatic stage before an individual is prompted to seek medical attention; indeed, it involves seeking out asymptomatic individuals among people who are not receiving medical attention for the disorder in question. The early detection of disease is worthwhile only for disorders that lend themselves to effective intervention and hence prevention. The identification of either trivial or untreatable conditions can cause anxiety with no useful result and would therefore not be appropriate for screening. Often screening is carried out to select individuals for a diagnostic test. The screening may take the form of a simple enquiry such as determining the age of a pregnant woman when screening for Down's syndrome (so that older women can be offered the diagnostic test, amniocentesis), or it may take the form of a special test such as maternal serum alpha-fetoprotein estimation when screening for neural tube defects.

The performance of screening tests as well as diagnostic tests involves three important measures (or parameters): (i) the detection rate (DR), (ii) the false-positive rate (FPR) and (iii) the odds of being affected given a positive result (OAPR).

The **detection rate** (or **sensitivity**) **of a test** (DR) is the proportion of affected individuals with positive test results (Table 8).

The **false-positive rate of a test (FPR)** is the proportion of unaffected individuals with positive test results (Table 8).

The **odds of being affected given a positive result (OAPR)** is the ratio of the number of affected individuals among those with positive test results, i.e. true positives : false positives.

The FPR of a test is sometimes expressed as the specificity, which is the FPR as a percentage subtracted from 100%, for example, an FPR of 3% is the same as a specificity of 97%.

As measures of screening performance, the DR and FPR have the important advantage that they are independent of disease prevalence. Hence estimates from one population can be applied to others. The odds of being affected given a positive result, however, does depend on the prevalence of the disorder being tested for.

Table 8 provides an algebraic description of the DR and FPR for a test with qualitative (or categorical) results. Some tests, such as cervical smear examinations for cancer of the cervix or karyotype determinations for chromosomal abnormality, are naturally categorical. Other tests, such as the maternal serum alpha-fetoprotein measurement for spina bifida screening, yield results as a continuous variable. In such cases, the DR and FPR depend on the screening cut-off level used to distinguish positive from negative results. These rates can be determined from the relative frequency distributions of the screening variable for affected and unaffected subjects. For example, the cut-off level A in Figure 8 will have a DR given by the area under the curve for affected subjects to the right of cut-off level A, and the FPR will be given by the area under the curve for unaffected subjects to the right of the same cut-off level. In this example, the higher the cut-off level (say, B or C) the lower the DR and the lower the FPR.

Table 8

Algebraic summary of detection and false-positive rates of a qualitative test

Test result	Affected	Unaffected	Total
Positive	a	b	a+b
Negative	c	d	c+d
Total	a+c	b+d	a+b+c+d

Detection rate (sensitivity) = $\dfrac{a}{a+c}$

False-positive rate (1 – specificity) = $\dfrac{b}{b+d}$

a are true positives   b are false positives
c are false negatives   d are true negatives

The detection rate and the false-positive rate are independent of disease prevalence

A screening flow diagram can be helpful – such as the one in Figure 9 illustrating the effect of using a test with an 80% DR and a 4% FPR when screening for a disorder with a prevalence of 1%. The OAPR after the screening test is 1:5, and 38:1 after using a diagnostic test with a DR of 95% and an FPR of 0.5%. If the prevalence of the disorder were 0.5%, the OAPRs would be halved to 1:10 and 19:1 respectively. This shows how the prevalence of the disorder being screened for has an important

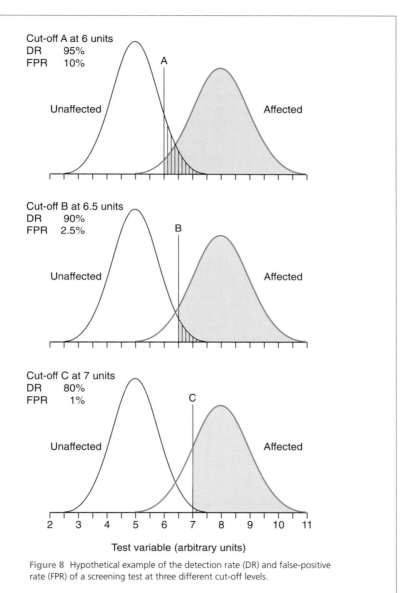

Cut-off A at 6 units
DR   95%
FPR   10%

A

Unaffected   Affected

Cut-off B at 6.5 units
DR   90%
FPR   2.5%

B

Unaffected   Affected

Cut-off C at 7 units
DR   80%
FPR   1%

C

Unaffected   Affected

2   3   4   5   6   7   8   9   10   11

Test variable (arbitrary units)

Figure 8 Hypothetical example of the detection rate (DR) and false-positive rate (FPR) of a screening test at three different cut-off levels.

influence on the results of screening. The more common the disorder, the more likely it is that a positive test result will be associated with that disorder, so that with a common disorder a screening test with a relatively poor DR and FPR might be acceptable, but not if the disorder were rarer.

The OAPR can be expressed as a probability, i.e. 'true positives/all positives' instead of 'true positive:false positives'. This is known as the positive predictive value (PPV): 80:400 = 1:5, which is equivalent to $1/(1 + 5) = 1/6 \cong 17\%$ in our example. See Box 3. The OAPR is a more useful parameter than the PPV because it is numerically easier to compute when tests are performed in sequence (see Figure 9), and it provides a better impression of the relative performance of tests. In the example shown in Figure 9, the OAPR of 38:1 is equivalent to a PPV of 97% (38/39). If the DR of the screening test were only 40%, the OAPR would be reduced by half (19:1) but the PPV, 95% (19/20), only appears a little lower.

Box 3

OAPR and PPV

In a particular population being tested:

- **the odds of being affected given a positive result (OAPR)**
  = all true positives : all false-positives

- **the positive predictive value (PPV)**
  = all true positives/all positives (all true and all false)

The OAPR (or PPV) depends on disease prevalence as well as on the detection and false-positive rates

---

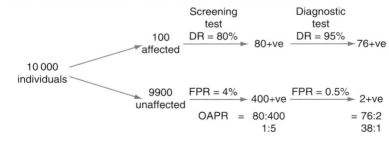

(The critical first step is to separate individuals into 'affected' and 'unaffected', not into screen-positive and screen-negative)

Figure 9 Flow chart to show the performance of screening and diagnostic tests.

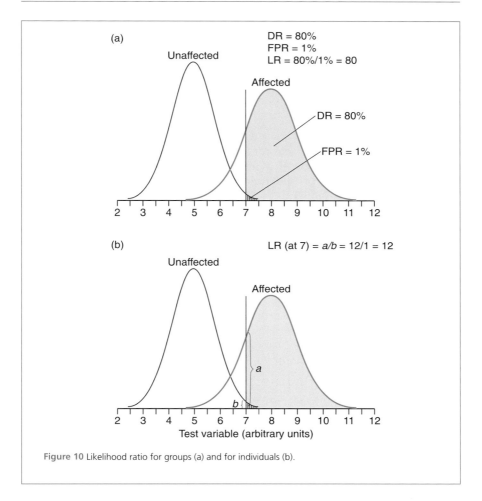

Figure 10 Likelihood ratio for groups (a) and for individuals (b).

The likelihood ratio

For groups of people, the **likelihood ratio** (LR) is the detection rate divided by the false-positive rate (DR/FPR) (see Figure 10a). This is the number of times individuals with positive results are more likely to have the disorder for which they are being tested compared with individuals who have not been tested.

The LR multiplied by the prevalence of the disorder (expressed as an odds) equals the OAPR. This is a useful way of calculating the OAPR. That is,

OAPR = LR × prevalence as an odds

So, for example (see Figure 10a), if the DR is 80% and the FPR is 1% then the LR is

80%/1%, or 80. If the prevalence of the disorder were 1 per 1000 (i.e. 1:999, which is nearly the same as 1000) then

$$\begin{aligned} \text{OAPR} &= 80 \times 1{:}1000 \\ &= 80{:}1000 \\ &= 1{:}1000/80 \\ &= 1{:}12.5 \end{aligned}$$

For *individuals* the LR is the height of the relative distribution curve for the affected individuals at the test value for that individual divided by the height of the curve for unaffected individuals at the same test value. So, for example, an individual with a test result of 7 (arbitrary units) in Figure 10b has an LR of 12, and

$$\begin{aligned} \text{OAPR} &= 12 \times 1{:}1000 \\ &= 12{:}1000 \\ &= 1{:}1000/12 \\ &= 1{:}83 \end{aligned}$$

A real example of using this calculation to determine the risk of a fatal stroke in a 70-year-old with a diastolic blood pressure of 105 mmHg is shown in Box 4.

Box 4

The risk of a man dying of a stroke at age 70 is about 20 per 10 000 per year (nearly equal to an odds ratio of 20:10 000). This information can be obtained from sources such as the ONS mortality tables (see Figure 11). Figure 12 shows the distributions of diastolic blood pressures in men who subsequently died from strokes and those who did not. The likelihood ratio (LR) for any individual is the ratio of the heights of the distribution curves at the individual's blood pressure. For a 70-year-old man with a diastolic blood pressure of 105 mmHg, the LR is about 3, so his risk becomes 3×20:10000=60:10000 or about 0.6%. Similarly, if a further screening test were carried out, for example measuring the man's serum cholesterol, then the results from this test could be combined to give an overall risk by again calculating the LR from distribution curves of stroke mortality and serum cholesterol levels and then multiplying the odds of 60:10000 by the new LR, assuming that diastolic blood pressure and cholesterol levels are independent, which is the case.

Requirements for a worthwhile screening programme

Before introducing screening, certain requirements need to be met. A knowledge of the disorder in question, including its prevalence and natural history, is needed to ensure that the disease is sufficiently common and serious to represent an important medical problem. An effective remedy must be available. The performance of the screening test should be known in terms of its detection and false-positive rates. The screening test must be simple, inexpensive, acceptable and

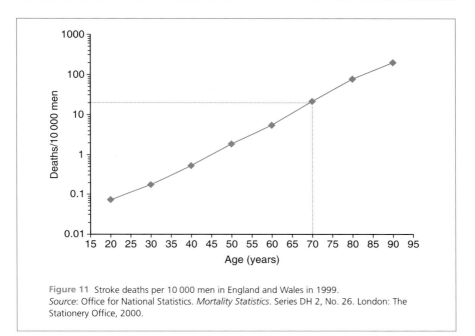

Figure 11 Stroke deaths per 10 000 men in England and Wales in 1999.
Source: Office for National Statistics. *Mortality Statistics*. Series DH 2, No. 26. London: The Stationery Office, 2000.

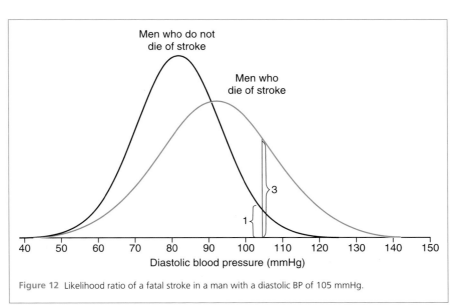

Figure 12 Likelihood ratio of a fatal stroke in a man with a diastolic BP of 105 mmHg.

safe, and facilities must be available to provide the screening service and consequent remedy. Equity of access to all who stand to gain from the screening programme, as well as equity in the quality of service provided, are important. It should be unacceptable to have one form of screening available in one part of the country but another elsewhere, unless there are good reasons for this, such as a marked difference in the prevalence of the disorder in different regions. The whole process from initial screening to application of the remedy must be ethical and regarded as desirable and one that offers value for money. Table 9 provides a summary of the requirements of a worthwhile screening programme and Table 10 lists examples that, in general, meet these requirements. Worthwhile screening programmes can, of course, fail through being badly implemented.

The requirements of a worthwhile screening test for a **cancer** pose special difficulties. It can be difficult to determine whether screening for a particular cancer and starting early treatment improves prognosis by delaying or preventing death from the cancer. In the past, *survival* (the time between initial diagnosis and death) has been misleadingly measured as an end-point. This is subject to two important biases. First, any method of achieving an earlier diagnosis will increase survival even if the date of death is unchanged: this prolongation between diagnosis and death is called *lead time bias*. The second bias arises because cancer screening involves periodic examinations, say every three years. Screening will detect more slowly growing tumours, because rapidly growing tumours are more likely to develop and proceed to clinical presentation within the interval between two consecutive screening examinations. The survival of such slowly growing screen-detected cancers will inevitably be greater than average. This is an example of biased sampling; it has been given the term *length time bias*.

Effective screening must prolong survival, but because of these two biases prolonged survival alone is insufficient evidence that screening genuinely affects prognosis. Both biases can be avoided by using *mortality* from the specific cancer (death rate, the number of deaths from cancer at a given age divided by the number of people at risk) as an end-point instead of survival. Mortality measures death rates whereas survival measures time to death from a given starting point. Mortality is not subject to lead time bias or length time bias, but survival is subject to both.

Mortality could be subject to bias if individuals who were screened were at higher (or lower) risk of developing the cancer in question than those not screened. If women of higher social class were more likely to be screened for cervical cancer, for example, mortality in screened women would tend to be lower than expected, regardless of the efficacy of screening. The only way of reliably avoiding such selection bias is to randomise individuals to screened and control groups and compare the death rates from the cancer in question in these two groups, i.e. to carry out a randomised controlled trial (see pages 20–24). One can then be sure that one is comparing like with like.

Table 9

Requirements for a worthwhile screening programme

1.	Disorder	Well defined
2.	Prevalence	Known
3.	Natural history	Medically important disorder
4.	Remedy*	An effective remedy or treatment is available
5.	Financial	Cost-effective
6.	Facilities	Available or easily installed
7.	Acceptability	Procedures following a positive result are generally agreed and acceptable both to the screening authorities and to the patients
8.	Equity	Equal access to screening services
9.	Test	Simple and safe
10.	Test performance*	Detection rate and false-positive rate known and acceptable. For a quantitative screening test, the distributions of test values in affected and unaffected individuals should be known, the extent of overlap sufficiently small, and a suitable cut-off level defined

*For a disease, such as cancer, in which the number of cases in the population at the time of screening is unknown (so the detection rate is always unknown because of this), the combined effect of screening and treatment should be known in terms of the proportional reduction in mortality from that disease arising from screening, usually determined from the results of randomised trials.

Table 10

Examples of worthwhile screening

Disorder	Initial screening test or enquiry	Subsequent test	Approximate proportion preventable
Antenatal screening			
Down's syndrome	Quadruple test (maternal age serum AFP, hCG, uE$_3$ and inhibin A)	Amniocentesis (karyotype)	80%
Open neural tube defects (anencephaly and spina bifida)	Maternal serum AFP	Amniotic fluid alpha-fetoprotein, acetylcholinesterase and/or ultrasound	90%
β-Thalassaemia	Red cell mean corpuscular volume	Haemoglobin electrophoresis, DNA analysis	95%
Neonatal screening			
Congenital hypothyroidism (cretinism)	Serum TSH and/or thyroxine	Repeat screening tests	95%
Phenylketonuria	Serum phenylalanine	Repeat screening tests and serum tyrosine	95%
Adult screening			
Mortality from:			
Cancer of the cervix	Cervical smear (≥ 25 years)	Repeat smears and colposcopy	80%
Cancer of the breast	Mammography (≥ 50 years)	Further mammography	30%
Cancer of the colon or rectum	Faecal occult blood (≥ 60 years)	Colonoscopy	15%
Abdominal aortic aneurysms	Ultrasound (≥ 65 years)		50%
Diabetic retinopathy	Identify diabetics	Retinal fundoscopy or photographic examination	60%

Patterns of births, mortality and morbidity

A useful description of the patterns of births, mortality and morbidity in a country can often be obtained from national organisations concerned with the collection of vital statistics. Appendix I lists some sources of these statistics. The Office for National Statistics and similar offices in other countries play a crucial role in providing the data needed for determining public health policy and the appropriate allocation of resources for medical care.

Population of England and Wales

The population of England and Wales in 2000 was about 53 million and that of Great Britain (England, Wales and Scotland) was 58 million. If everyone in England and Wales lived for 100 years and the age distribution was uniform, there would be 530 000 deaths each year. In reality, the age at death is lower and the number of deaths higher (about 540 000 per year).

The age and sex distributions of the population are shown in Figure 13. Up to age 45, there are more males than females; above age 50, the effect of the higher mortality in men is apparent and the number of females exceeds males. Over the age of 85, about three-quarters of the population are women. The smaller number of people aged 0–4 (3 168 000) than 30–34 (4 211 000) reflects the falling birth rate.

Birth rate and induced abortion rate

The *birth rate* is the number of live births and stillbirths in a given year divided by the estimated total population at the middle of the year. For England and Wales in 2000, it was 11.4 per 1000. This rate corresponds to an average of 1.7 babies born to each woman (the total fertility rate). A value of slightly above 2.0 is needed to maintain population numbers. The induced abortion rate at present is about one-fifth of the birth rate. The variation in the proportion of pregnancies that end in an induced (so-called 'legal') abortion between different countries is shown in Figure 14.

Perinatal and infant mortality

The *stillbirth rate* is the number of stillbirths divided by the total number of births. The term *stillbirth* in England and Wales applies to any infant born after the 24th week of pregnancy and showing no signs of life after birth. The rate in 2001 was 5.3

per thousand total births. The *perinatal mortality rate* is the number of stillbirths plus deaths in the first week of life divided by total births. The rate in England and Wales in 2001 was 8.0 per thousand total births. The *infant mortality rate* is the number of deaths in live-born infants under one year of age divided by total live births. This was 5.4 per thousand live births in 2001.

In summary, about 0.5% of babies are stillborn, 0.25% of liveborn babies die in the first week of life and another 0.25% die between the 2nd and 52nd weeks of life.

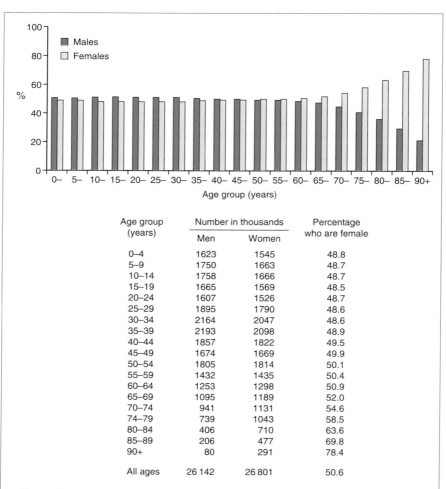

Age group (years)	Number in thousands		Percentage who are female
	Men	Women	
0–4	1623	1545	48.8
5–9	1750	1663	48.7
10–14	1758	1666	48.7
15–19	1665	1569	48.5
20–24	1607	1526	48.7
25–29	1895	1790	48.6
30–34	2164	2047	48.6
35–39	2193	2098	48.9
40–44	1857	1822	49.5
45–49	1674	1669	49.9
50–54	1805	1814	50.1
55–59	1432	1435	50.4
60–64	1253	1298	50.9
65–69	1095	1189	52.0
70–74	941	1131	54.6
74–79	739	1043	58.5
80–84	406	710	63.6
85–89	206	477	69.8
90+	80	291	78.4
All ages	26 142	26 801	50.6

Figure 13 Percentage of males and females in each 5-year age band, England and Wales, 2000. *Source*: Office for National Statistics. *Mortality Statistics*. Series DH2, No. 27. London: The Stationery Office, 2000.

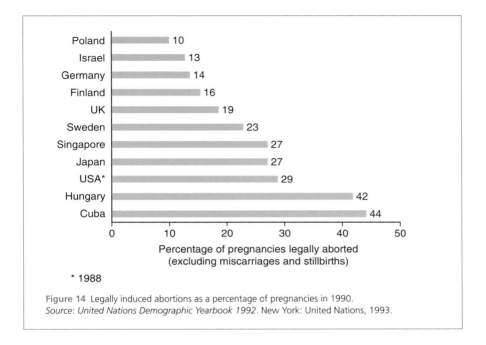

* 1988

Figure 14 Legally induced abortions as a percentage of pregnancies in 1990.
Source: United Nations Demographic Yearbook 1992. New York: United Nations, 1993.

Mortality

The introduction of death registration was a landmark in the development of epidemiology. It permitted the quantitative assessment of the frequency of fatal disease, both over time and between different geographical regions. Britain was one of the first countries to collect mortality statistics routinely, and annual figures have been produced since 1838–39. Later, death registration providing details of the cause of death was introduced. The importance of accurate death certification, when necessary incorporating autopsy information, cannot be underestimated. It is important in relation to nearly all epidemiological and public health activities as well as the obvious importance in clinical medicine of knowing the cause of death. Appendix II gives an example of a death certificate together with guidance on how one should be completed and interpreted. Figure 15a shows that the death rate fell steeply from the middle of the 19th century and Figure 15b shows that infant mortality has fallen rapidly from the beginning of the 20th century. Figures 16a and 16b show the reduction in selected age-specific death rates from 1841 to 1995. There has been a fall in all age groups, with the greatest percentage reductions being among younger people. For example, in persons aged 25–34 years, there has been a 90% reduction in mortality, compared with a reduction of 47% in those aged 75–84 years. The main reason for the fall in mortality in the young has been the decline in

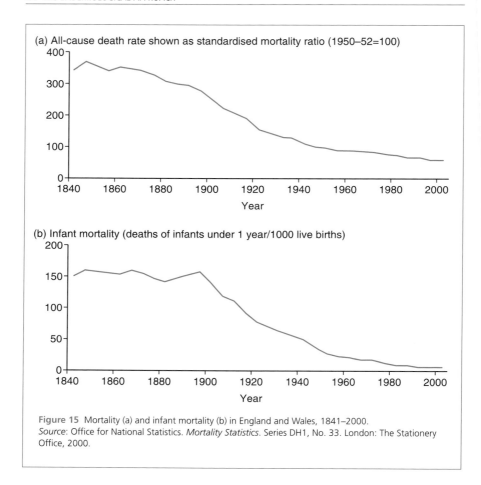

Figure 15 Mortality (a) and infant mortality (b) in England and Wales, 1841–2000.
Source: Office for National Statistics. *Mortality Statistics*. Series DH1, No. 33. London: The Stationery Office, 2000.

infectious diseases. Figure 16a shows mortality plotted on an arithmetic scale, in which a constant slope indicates a constant absolute change in the number of deaths from year to year. The steeper downward slope in the older age groups shows that the absolute number of deaths changed more in older people than in younger ones. Figure 16b shows the same data plotted on a logarithmic (proportional) scale, in which a constant slope indicates a constant proportional change in the number of deaths. This illustrates more clearly the greater proportional decline in mortality in younger people. (It is important to identify which scale is used when interpreting graphs.) Figure 17a shows the fall in the standardised mortality ratio for tuberculosis from about 1500 in the mid-1850s to below 10 in recent years. Most of this reduction occurred well before the introduction of specific medical interventions such as the use of antibiotics and immunisation or the use of special investigative techniques such as X-ray. It has instead been largely due to the improvement in living standards, particularly in housing conditions and nutrition. (Figure 17b shows the same data used in Figure 17a on a logarithmic (proportional) scale; this shows more clearly the increase in the proportional rate of fall in mortality from tuberculosis after about 1945 – a change that was probably the result of antibiotics and BCG vaccination, which in effect accelerated the underlying trend.)

With the reduction in age-specific death rates, particularly in childhood, the

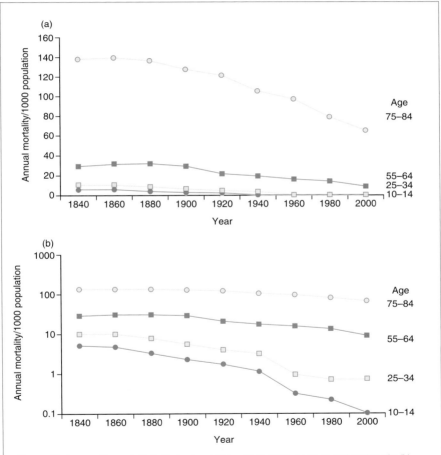

Figure 16 Age-specific mortality in England and Wales, 1841–2000: (a) on an arithmetic scale; (b) on a logarithmic (proportional) scale.
Source: Office for National Statistics. *Mortality Statistics*. Series DH1, No. 33. London: The Stationery Office, 2000.

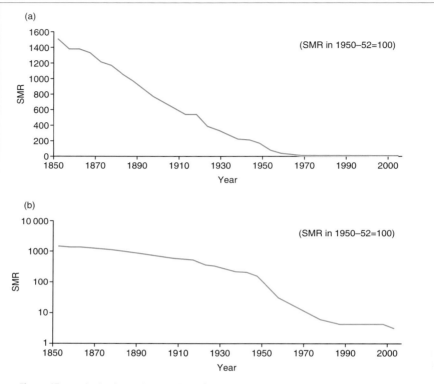

Figure 17 Standardised mortality ratio (SMR) from tuberculosis in England and Wales, 1851–2000: (a) on an arithmatic scale; (b) on a logarithmic (proportional) scale.
Source: Office for National Statistics. *Mortality Statistics*. Series DH2, No.27. London: The Stationery Office, 2000.

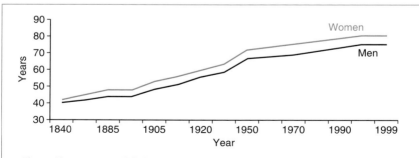

Figure 18 Expectation of life from birth in England and Wales, 1840–1999.
Source: Office for National Statistics. *Mortality Statistics*. Series DH1, No. 33. London: The Stationery Office, 2000.

expectation of life has increased. From birth, it is now about 80 years in women and 75 in men, compared with 42 and 40 respectively around 1850 (see Figure 18). Not surprisingly, therefore, most deaths occur between the ages of 75 and 84 (see Figure 19).

The major causes of death vary considerably according to age. The main causes in the first four weeks of life are those associated with prematurity, congenital malformations and complications of birth. The main causes of death during the remaining part of the first year of life are congenital malformations and sudden infant death syndrome (infectious disease and respiratory disorders are also significant causes of death in the first year). Table 11 shows the age-specific death rates in 2000 in England and Wales for selected causes of death and Figure 20 shows how the major causes of death differ in different age groups.

Table 11 shows that at every age males have a higher mortality than females. The death rate in the first year of life is similar to the death rate of people aged about 55. The lowest death rates are seen at age 5–14; thereafter they increase throughout life. The annual risk of dying from any cause exceeds about 1% in men from the age of about 60 and in women from the age of about 65.

Accidents are the major cause of death in both children (1–14 years) and young adults (15–34 years), with road traffic accidents representing about one-third of these. In adults aged 35–54 years, for both sexes combined, cancer is the major cause of death, followed by ischaemic heart disease and cerebrovascular disease. Two diseases have increased rapidly during most of the 20th century, namely ischaemic heart disease and lung cancer, both of which are more common in men than in women. The rise in lung cancer mortality during the 20th century (Figure 21) is particularly striking, not only on account of its magnitude but also because it is

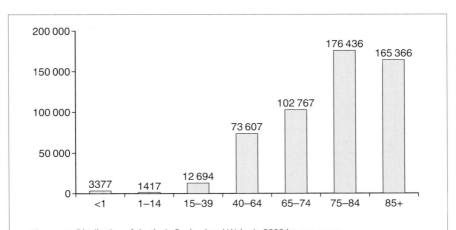

Figure 19 Distribution of deaths in England and Wales in 2000 by age group.
Source: Office for National Statistics. *Mortality Statistics*. Series DH2, No. 27. London: The Stationery Office, 2000.

Table 11

Death rates per million population from selected causes by age and sex in England and Wales in 2000

Cause	Sex	<1	1–4	5–14	15–24	25–34	35–44	45–54	55–64	65–74	75–84	>84
All causes	M	6 091	256	143	641	925	1 493	3 842	10 392	29 762	76 077	181 330
	F	5 057	197	101	275	440	988	2 610	6 409	18 181	50 948	147 640
Lung cancer	M	—	—	—	1	4	35	268	1 114	3 075	5 306	5 491
	F	—	—	—	0	2	31	191	612	1 579	2 102	1 575
Breast cancer	F	—	—	—	2	37	160	444	721	992	1 577	2 592
Colorectal cancer	M	—	—	—	2	5	24	119	433	1 152	2 212	3 188
	F	—	—	—	3	5	25	90	253	642	1 341	2 292
Other cancers	M	6	36	33	48	92	211	820	2 439	6 237	12 665	21 159
	F	14	29	25	38	81	216	672	1 697	3 705	6 607	9 559
Ischaemic heart disease	M	—	1	—	2	24	187	893	2 824	8 072	18 969	36 300
	F	—	1	0	0	6	45	189	784	3 352	10 533	24 798
Cerebrovascular disease	M	32	3	3	6	20	59	177	469	1 914	6 958	18 932
	F	10	2	2	6	15	45	148	358	1 483	6 381	21 608
Other circulatory disease	M	55	7	3	20	40	82	238	677	2 339	6 634	16 344
	F	78	18	4	16	26	53	125	393	1 488	5 012	15 403
Accidents, injury etc	M	107	45	50	398	478	438	392	350	436	947	2 992
	F	115	33	18	109	108	133	153	156	252	698	2 515
Chronic obstructive airways disease	M	—	4	3	7	8	15	79	436	1 784	5 250	10 047
	F	—	—	3	5	7	14	64	305	1 264	2 686	3 479

Source: Office for National Statistics. *Mortality Statistics.* Series DH2, No. 27. London: The Stationery Office, 2000.

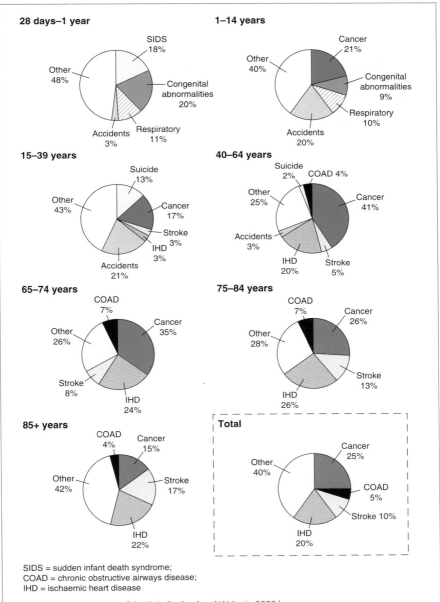

SIDS = sudden infant death syndrome;
COAD = chronic obstructive airways disease;
IHD = ischaemic heart disease

Figure 20 Main causes of death in England and Wales in 2000 by age group.
Source: Office for National Statistics. *Mortality Statistics*. Series DH2, No. 27. London: The Stationery Office, 2000.

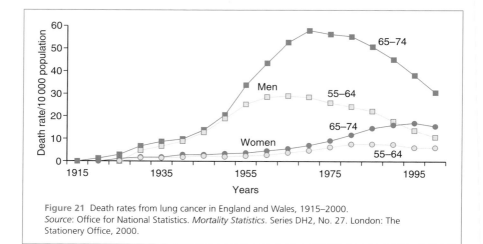

Figure 21 Death rates from lung cancer in England and Wales, 1915–2000. *Source:* Office for National Statistics. *Mortality Statistics.* Series DH2, No. 27. London: The Stationery Office, 2000.

almost all caused by smoking. Some of the early increase must have been due to improvements in diagnosis (lung cancer up to the mid-1900s may have been misdiagnosed as TB) but the differences in lung cancer mortality between the sexes indicate that this alone could not explain the rise. In the last quarter of the 20th century, lung cancer death rates declined in men because of a decline in smoking and a switch to lower-tar cigarettes. There was also a decline in death rates from ischaemic heart disease in both sexes, mainly due to improvements in treatment.

Taking men and women of all ages together, about 20% of deaths are caused by ischaemic heart disease, 25% by cancer, 10% by strokes and 5% by chronic obstructive airways disease, leaving 40% attributable to other causes (Figure 20). The distribution of cancer deaths according to the organ in which the cancer originated is shown in Figure 22.

Figure 23 and Table 12 show the UK AIDS figures, demonstrating the relatively low mortality from this disease in the UK up to December 2000 and the improved efficacy of treatments. The future of the epidemic in the UK remains uncertain, but it does not look as if it will increase.

Epidemiological modelling can be useful in predicting future trends in the incidence of a disease. A recent important example is the prediction of mortality from malignant mesothelioma in British men in relation to UK asbestos imports. Imports of asbestos rose to a peak in the 1960s and 1970s. Mesothelioma develops usually decades after the exposure to asbestos (the average interval is about 50 years) (Figure 24). Exposure in young men is therefore important; men exposed in older age will die of other causes first. As a result, the lifetime probability of dying from mesothelioma for British men has increased from almost zero in men born around 1900 to about 1% for men born around 1950. There will be over 3000

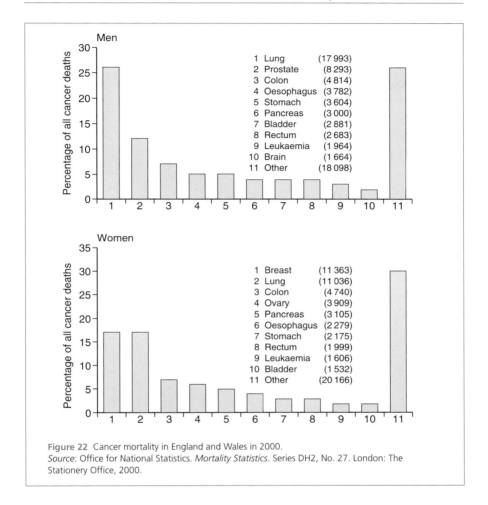

Figure 22 Cancer mortality in England and Wales in 2000.
Source: Office for National Statistics. *Mortality Statistics*. Series DH2, No. 27. London: The Stationery Office, 2000.

deaths a year from this disease in about 2020, while in 1970 there were only 200 – an epidemic that will only disappear when all persons exposed to asbestos have died. (In 2001, there were 1577 deaths from mesothelioma in England and Wales, which is close to the number predicted.)

Statistics on cause of death are collected from death certificates. An example of a death certificate with notes on how to complete one is given in Appendix II.

Differences in mortality between the sexes

In England and Wales during 2000, the death rate was 9.0 per 1000 for men and 10.0 per 1000 for women, which means that 0.9% of men died and 1.0% of women died.

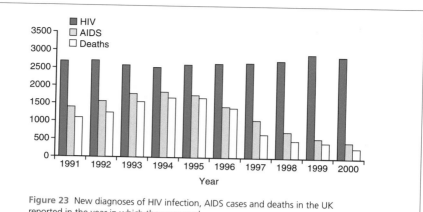

Figure 23 New diagnoses of HIV infection, AIDS cases and deaths in the UK reported in the year in which they occurred.
Source: AIDS and HIV infection in the United Kingdom: monthly report – January 2002. *Communicable Disease Report*, Vol 12, No. 5, 31 January 2002.

Table 12

HIV-infected individuals by year of first reported UK diagnosis: UK data to end-December 2000

How infection was probably acquired	1985	1990	1995	2000
Sex between men	2105	1691	1466	1429
Sex between men and women (total)	54	534	848	1867
Injecting drug use (IDU)	277	198	182	101
Blood factor treatment (e.g. for haemophilia)	664	4	4	3
Blood/tissue transfer (e.g. transfusion)	22	20	16	19
Mother to infant	3	29	59	91
Other/undetermined	98	57	61	144
Total	3223	2533	2636	3654

Table 11 (top two rows) shows that at each age the death rate is 20–70% higher in males than females.

There are 105 boys born for every 100 girls. This small excess is slowly reduced by mortality until at age 50 there are equal numbers of women and men (see Figure 13). Among elderly people, the ratio of women to men increases dramatically, and is 1.2:1 at age 70, 1.6:1 at 80 and 4:1 at 90; among people reaching 100 (about 1500 a year), the sex ratio is 10:1. The preponderance of elderly women occurs because mortality from many diseases

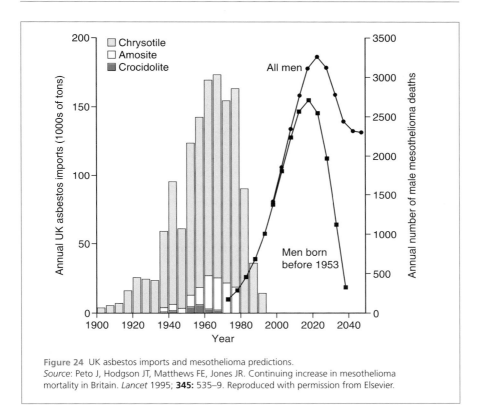

Figure 24 UK asbestos imports and mesothelioma predictions.
Source: Peto J, Hodgson JT, Matthews FE, Jones JR. Continuing increase in mesothelioma mortality in Britain. *Lancet* 1995; **345**: 535–9. Reproduced with permission from Elsevier.

is higher in men, as shown in Table 11; the death of servicemen in the two world wars was a minor factor. The conditions that contribute most to the shorter life expectancy of men are ischaemic heart disease, lung cancer, stomach cancer, chronic bronchitis and emphysema, and, especially in young adults, trauma. The disparity in death rates between the sexes is explained in part by the differences in their habits (e.g. smoking) and occupation (e.g. work-related accidents), but this does not account for all of it.

Elderly people

About 19% (8.4 million) of the current population of England and Wales are aged 65 and over (16% of men, 22% of women). In Victorian times, this proportion was only 5%. Future projections (Figure 25) show that there will be even more old people, with fewer young people to care for them. An increase from 3 to 4 million aged over 75 is expected in the next 30–40 years. This has important consequences for public spending, as the elderly are heavy consumers of health and social services, and the prevalence of age-related diseases like Alzheimer's disease will increase.

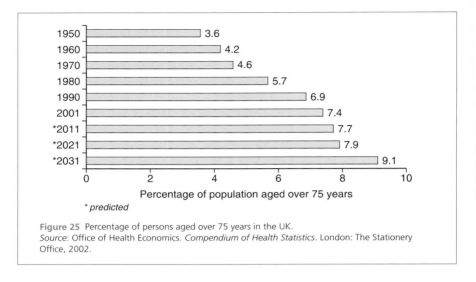

Figure 25 Percentage of persons aged over 75 years in the UK.
Source: Office of Health Economics. *Compendium of Health Statistics*. London: The Stationery Office, 2002.

Social and ethnic groups

Social class

In all societies, there are inequalities in health. Figure 26 shows the death rates in men in England and Wales classified according to social class – the system of categorising the population according to occupation that was devised by the Registrar General in 1875. There are five social classes (excluding the armed forces), one of which is divided into two subclasses. These are, as percentages of the population:

I	professional	5%
II	semi-professional	18%
IIIN	skilled non-manual	12%
IIIM	skilled manual	38%
IV	semi-skilled	18%
V	unskilled	9%

The differences in mortality among social classes illustrate the extent to which mortality rates in Western countries depend on lifestyle and environmental factors. Figure 26 shows that the mortality rate in social class V is about three times greater than that in social class I. For accidents in children under 14 years of age, the difference is over eightfold. Nearly all diseases are more common in social classes IV and V than in classes I and II. For example, there are large differences in mortality from ischaemic heart disease and lung cancer, reflecting differences in smoking habit and diet between the social classes. A few diseases, however, are more common in social classes I and II. For example, breast cancer, multiple sclerosis, malignant

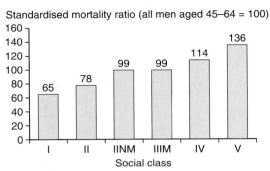

Figure 26 Mortality by social class, men aged 45–64 years in England and Wales. *Source*: Goldblatt P. Mortality by social class. 1971–85. In: *Population Trends*, No. 56. London: HMSO, 1989.

melanoma and Hodgkin's disease are more common in the professional occupations than in the unskilled. This observation suggests aetiological hypotheses – for example, the link between melanoma and sudden episodes of sunbathing among fair-skinned persons able to afford holidays in the sun and the loss of the protective effect of early pregnancy and multiparity in relation to breast cancer among women who delay having children and limit their family size.

From 2001, all official statistics and surveys have used a revised social class classification system called the National Statistics Socio-economic Classification (NS-SEC):

1. Higher managerial and professional occupations
2. Lower managerial and professional occupations
3. Intermediate occupations
4. Small employers and own-account workers
5. Lower supervisory and technical occupations
6. Semi-routine occupations
7. Routine occupations
8. Never worked and long-term unemployed

Minority ethnic groups

In 2000, the British population included a total of 4.1 million non-whites (Table 13). The ethnic minority populations are young – only 3% are aged over 65, compared with 16% of whites. Those of South Asian (Indian sub-continent) origin have a high mortality from ischaemic heart disease. Afro-Caribbeans have a comparatively low mortality from ischaemic heart disease, but high mortality from stroke, renal insufficiency and other blood pressure-related diseases.

Table 13

Ethnic minority groups in Great Britain in 2000

Ethnic group	Number	% of total population
Indian	1 000 000	1.8
Pakistani	700 000	1.2
Bangladeshi	300 000	0.5
Black Caribbean	500 000	0.9
Black African	400 000	0.7
Black other	300 000	0.5
Chinese	100 000	0.2
Other minorities	800 000	1.4
Total minorities	4 100 000	7.2
White	53 000 000	92.8
Total population	57 100 000	100

Source: Office for National Statistics. *Social Trends*, No. 32. London: The Stationery Office, 2002.

Regional variation in mortality

Figure 27 shows the standardised mortality ratios for different regions in England and Wales. The 'North–South' divide can be seen: mortality rates are higher in the North. This is not simply due to social class difference – the same North–South difference can be seen in each social class examined separately. Of the more common causes of death, those showing the greatest degree of regional variation are lung cancer and stomach cancer, chronic obstructive airways disease, ischaemic heart disease, and stroke. Both regional and social class variations are likely to reflect mainly differences in lifestyle (especially smoking) rather than access to medical treatment. The striking variation in mortality from ischaemic heart disease around the world is illustrated in Figure 28.

Morbidity

There are five main sources of information on the extent of illness in the population: (i) hospital statistics on the number of episodes of hospital illness and bed occupancy rates (counted as discharges from hospital and deaths in hospital); (ii) registration of all newly diagnosed cases of cancer; (iii) general practitioner consultation rates; (iv) self-reported illness in population surveys; and (v) statistics on infectious disease from the Public Health Laboratory Service (PHLS).

Figure 29 shows bed occupancy rates according to disease. Mental illness and mental handicap alone account for about 40% of all inpatient hospital days, mainly

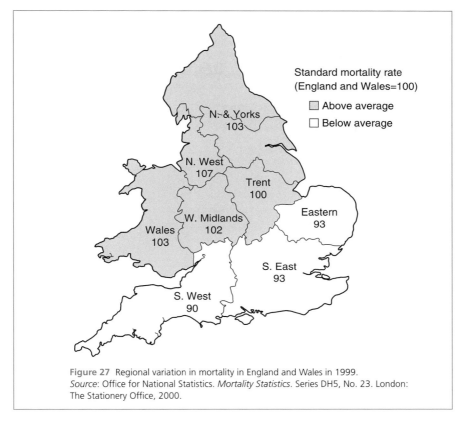

Figure 27 Regional variation in mortality in England and Wales in 1999.
Source: Office for National Statistics. *Mortality Statistics*. Series DH5, No. 23. London:
The Stationery Office, 2000.

because these admissions tend to be long-term. This represents a little-recognised but major health care commitment. Figure 30 shows the general practitioner consultation rates according to major disease groups. Consultation rates are higher for women than for men for nearly all conditions; overall, there were about 3.5 visits per person per year in 1991–92.

Figure 31 shows the main causes of blindness in England and Wales in 1990–91. One of the commonest causes among younger adults (16–64 years) is as a complication of diabetes (diabetic retinopathy), an occurrence that can largely be prevented in many cases by screening and early intervention (Rohan et al, 1989) (see Table 10).

It is not generally appreciated that up to about 1998 there was a substantial increase in the incidence of food poisoning in the UK, and the rate remains high. About 4.5 million cases occur in the UK each year, with 1 in 6 resulting in a visit to a doctor (Donaldson, 2002). This represents about 8% of the population being affected each year. Figure 32 shows the trend between 1986 and 2000 based on

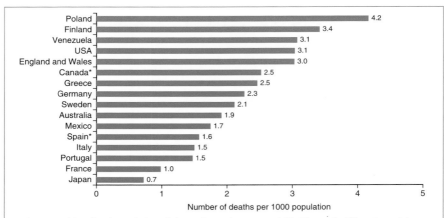

Figure 28 Mortality due to ischaemic heart disease in men aged 55–64 years in different countries in 1999 (*1998).
Source: WHO 2002. http://www3.who.int/whosis/mort/

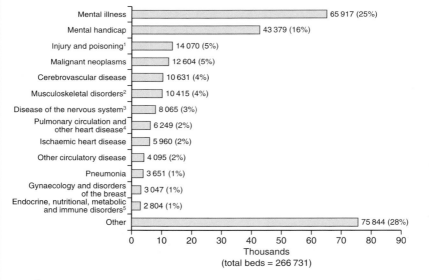

[1] Includes 4052 beds/day for fractured neck of femur
[2] Includes arthropathies and back and joint disorders
[3] Includes Parkinsons's disease (1119), cerebral palsy (1193), epilepsy (1675) and multiple sclerosis (965)
[4] Heart failure accounts for 3011 beds/day
[5] Diabetes mellitus accounts for 1536 beds/day

Figure 29 Average daily hospital bed use in England in 1992–93.
Source: Department of Health. *Hospital Episode Statistics*, Vol 1: *England, Financial Year 1992–93.* London: HMSO.

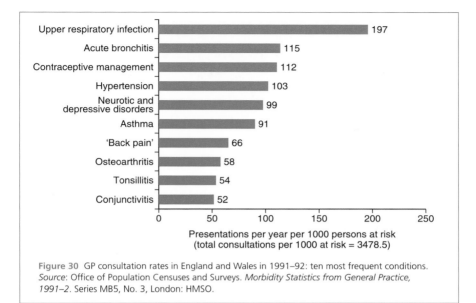

Figure 30 GP consultation rates in England and Wales in 1991–92: ten most frequent conditions. *Source*: Office of Population Censuses and Surveys. *Morbidity Statistics from General Practice, 1991–2.* Series MB5, No. 3, London: HMSO.

laboratory isolations notified to the Public Health Laboratory Service. There was a 500% increase in such notifications. Food poisoning due to *Campylobacter* has particularly increased over the period. These notifications substantially underestimate the incidence of food poisoning, but the changes over time probably provide a reasonably accurate indication of trends. It is important to be aware that

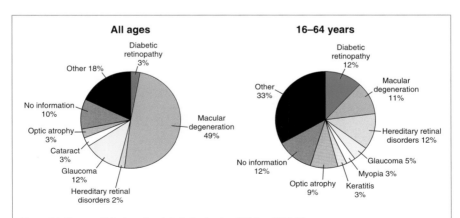

Figure 31 Causes of blindness in adults in England and Wales, 1990–91. *Source*: Office of Population Censuses and Surveys. *Studies on Medical and Population Subjects*, 1990–1. SMPS, No. 57. London: HMSO.

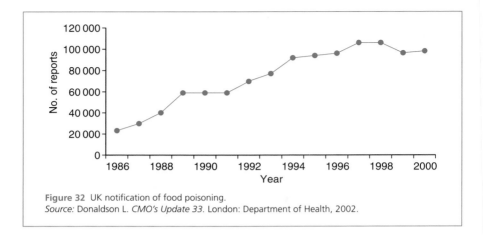

Figure 32 UK notification of food poisoning.
Source: Donaldson L. *CMO's Update 33*. London: Department of Health, 2002.

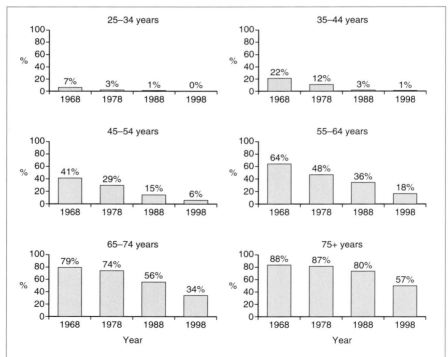

Figure 33 Percentage of adults with no natural teeth in England and Wales, 1968–98, according to age.
Source: Steele JG, Treasure E, Pitts NB et al. Total tooth loss in the United Kingdom in 1998 and implications for the future. *Br Dent J* 2000; **189:** 598–603.

food poisoning is not simply a problem associated with economically poor countries. It requires substantial vigilance and control over the manufacture and preparation of food, both in catering establishments and in the home. The key to avoiding food poisoning is strict adherence to principles of good hygiene.

One of the less well known, but important, public health achievements of recent decades has been in the area of preventive dentistry. Figure 33 shows the proportion of adults with no natural teeth in England and Wales between 1968 and 1998; in persons aged 45–54 years, 40% were without their own teeth in 1968, but by 1998 this proportion had fallen to 6%. This advance in dental health has principally arisen from the widespread use of fluoridated toothpaste (in 1969, only 2% of toothpaste was fluoridated, while now the proportion is about 95%), more effective and regular brushing of teeth, and a greater emphasis on the repair and retention of diseased teeth, rather than extraction.

The developing world

The above description of health in the UK is fairly typical of an economically rich Western nation. The pattern of disease in the developing world is quite different, but is becoming closer to that in so-called developed countries. Table 14 compares the ten leading causes of death in developed and developing countries – a breakdown of about 56 million deaths worldwide, 16 million from cardiovascular disease, which has become the leading cause of death in 'developing' countries (about one-sixth of deaths) as well as 'developed' countries (about one-third of deaths). Apart from malaria and certain disorders specific to particular regions, it is in many respects similar to that found in Britain in the early part of the 19th century, with infectious disease accounting for the major burden of mortality. Many diseases typically thought of as 'tropical', such as leprosy and onchocerciasis, account for relatively little mortality overall. Infant mortality rates in developing countries are typical of those seen in Britain over 100 years ago, some 10–20 times greater than those seen in the rich countries of the world today (Figure 34). Similarly, the expectation of life in developing countries is low – nearly half that seen in industrialised countries (see Figure 7).

Poverty is the main cause of disease in the economically poor countries of the world, where three-quarters of the world's six billion inhabitants live. This three-quarters of the world's population live on a fifth of its income. It has been estimated that improved water and sanitation would prevent 80% of deaths in the developing world. In addition to poverty-related diseases, some diseases typical of industrial countries are being exported to the poorer countries; a prime example is lung cancer, through the introduction of cigarette smoking, so that lung cancer, formerly a relatively rare cancer, is now the commonest fatal cancer in the world.

A useful way to compare the relative importance of various diseases in different countries is to calculate for each disease the years of life lost due to deaths from that

Table 14

Estimates of the ten leading causes of death in the world in 2000

World			Developed countries			Developing countries		
Rank	Cause	% of total deaths	Rank	Cause	% of total deaths	Rank	Cause	% of total deaths
1	Ischaemic heart disease	12.4	1	Ischaemic heart disease	22.6	1	Ischaemic heart disease	9.1
2	Cerebrovascular disease	9.2	2	Cerebrovascular disease	13.7	2	Cerebrovascular disease	8.0
3	Lower respiratory infections	6.9	3	Trachea, bronchus, lung cancers	4.5	3	Lower respiratory infections	7.7
4	HIV/AIDS	5.3	4	Lower respiratory infections	3.7	4	HIV/AIDS	6.9
5	COPD	4.5	5	COPD	3.1	5	Perinatal conditions	5.6
6	Perinatal conditions	4.4	6	Colon and rectum cancers	2.6	6	COPD	5.0
7	Diarrhoeal diseases	3.8	7	Stomach cancer	1.9	7	Diarrhoeal diseases	4.9
8	Tuberculosis	3.0	8	Self-inflicted injuries	1.9	8	Tuberculosis	3.7
9	Road traffic accidents	2.3	9	Diabetes	1.7	9	Malaria	2.6
10	Trachea, bronchus, lung	2.2	10	Breast cancer	1.6	10	Road traffic accidents	2.5

COPD = chronic obstructive pulmonary disease. Developed countries include European countries, former Soviet countries, Canada, USA, Japan, Australia and New Zealand.

Source: The World Health Report 2002. Geneva: World Health Organisation, 2002 (cited in Beaglehoe R, Yach D. Globalisation and the prevention and control of non-communicable disease: the neglected chronic diseases of adults. Lancet 2003; **362**: 903–8).

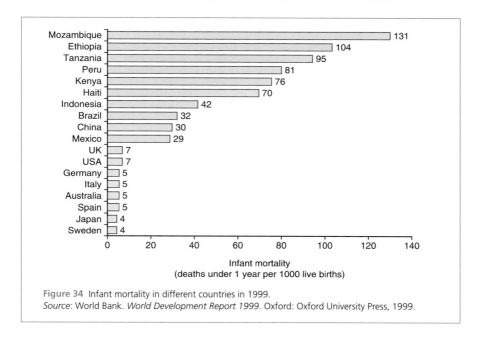

Figure 34 Infant mortality in different countries in 1999.
Source: World Bank. *World Development Report 1999.* Oxford: Oxford University Press, 1999.

particular disease. In this way, a disease that kills a person at age 60 results in a loss of fewer years of life than in a person who dies at, say, 20. Table 15 compares the years of life lost from three diseases that are important causes of mortality in the industrialised world (accidents, circulatory disease and cancer) with the years of life lost in the developing world. Sub-Saharan Africa and economically developed countries have been used for the comparison. While these three diseases account for 25% of years of life lost in Sub-Saharan Africa, they account for 73% in countries with established market economies. This is partly because life expectancy in Sub-Saharan Africa is about 50 years, compared with over 75 years in economically developed countries. But it also reflects differences in the age-specific incidence of these diseases in the different countries. The pattern of disease in the more developed countries has changed as we are able to live longer, and so are more likely to suffer from diseases occurring typically in old age. Table 16 shows the years of healthy life lost in Sub-Saharan Africa due to different diseases. Six groups of diseases account for 60% of life lost, namely diarrhoeal disease and malnutrition, measles, respiratory illness (mainly pneumonia), malaria, perinatal disorders, and HIV.

Diarrhoeal disease is one of the most important causes of morbidity and mortality in the developing world, where an estimated 500 million episodes of diarrhoea in children in Asia, Africa and Latin America in 1975 caused 5–18 million deaths. The problem is largely due to the vicious cycle that arises from contaminated water and

Table 15

Proportion of years of life lost due to accident, circulatory disease and cancer in economically developed countries and Sub-Saharan Africa in 1990

Cause of death	Percentage of years of life lost	
	Economically developed countries	Sub-Saharan Africa
Circulatory diseases	29	4
Cancer	24	3
Accidents (mainly road traffic)	20	18
Total	73	25

Source: Murray CJL, Lopez, AD (eds). *Global Burden of Disease* (http://www.hup.harvard.edu/catalog/MURGLO/html).

Table 16

Proportion of years of healthy life lost in Sub-Saharan Africa due to different diseases in 1990

Disease	Percentage
Diarrhoeal diseases and malnutrition	16
Respiratory illnesses, mainly pneumonia	13
Malaria	11
Measles	9
Perinatal disorders	8
HIV	3
Total	60

Source: Murray CJL, Lopez, AD (eds). *Global Burden of Disease* (http://www.hup.harvard.edu/catalog/MURGLO/html).

food and from malnutrition. Poorly nourished children are more liable to get diarrhoea and thereby infect others, who contaminate the water supplies. In Africa alone, 30% of children are estimated to be clinically underweight for their age, and 4% are seriously so with either kwashiorkor or marasmus (King, 1983).

The burden of disease from respiratory illness is largely due to the same infections that arise in industrialised countries – or did so before satisfactory control measures were introduced. They are mainly pneumonia, whooping cough, influenza, measles, TB and diphtheria. The difference between the developing world and the industrialised countries is not so much in the types of disease that occur but in the frequency and impact that they have.

Malaria is among the most serious health problems in many parts of tropical Africa: it is estimated to cause over one million deaths a year. Although other vector-borne diseases are less prominent than malaria in mortality and morbidity statistics, they are still significant. Two hundred million people have schistosomiasis (bilharzia) and another 200 million have filariasis. About a billion people in the developing world are infested by worms. Surveys in Sri Lanka, Bangladesh and Venezuela showed that over 90% of 6-year-old children were affected. The most common worm infestations are hookworm and roundworm (ascariasis).

Measles, while not a typical tropical disease, is an important cause of mortality in the developing world. This is partly due to reduced host defences in children suffering from malnutrition and other infections and to the fact that measles in the developing world occurs in infancy, when the complications of the disease are greater than at older ages. Perinatal disorders are largely those associated with prematurity, infections and congenital malformations. The HIV epidemic is having profound impacts on rates of infant, child and maternal mortality, on life expectancy and on economic growth, particularly in some parts of the developing world, notably Sub-Saharan Africa. Figure 35 shows the vast differences in the proportions of adults with HIV in different countries, ranging from 36% in Botswana to 0.1% in the UK and Germany. In Africa, there are now 16 countries in which more than one-tenth of the population is infected with HIV, and in most

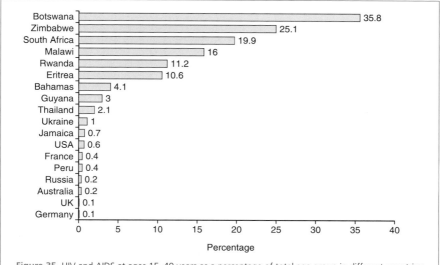

Figure 35 HIV and AIDS at ages 15–49 years as a percentage of total age group in different countries: estimates, 1999.
Source: Report on the Global HIV/AIDS epidemic – June 2000 (http://www.unaids.org/EN/resources/epidemiology.asp).

Sub-Saharan countries adults are acquiring HIV infection at a higher rate than ever before. Another problem in Africa is sickle-cell disease, which affects about 1 in 400 Africans; about 1 in 10 people of African descent carry the gene.

Within developing countries or regions, there are important geographical differences in the distribution of disease. These tend to reflect the local ecological conditions. For example, malaria is transmitted by certain kinds of mosquito and transmission of schistosomiasis depends on passage of the parasite from urine or faeces through certain kinds of water snail. Many parasitic diseases are restricted to certain locations.

Disease problems in the Third World cannot be solved by building hospitals, with their costly infrastructure of staff and equipment, which tend to be used by a privileged minority rather than the poor. Often little or no medical care is available for people who live in villages, where most of the world's poor live. The greatest need is for simple measures such as ensuring the supply and quality of food, the provision of clean water supplies and effective sewage, and the control of fertility. The WHO's programme for primary health care hopes to achieve this with the emphasis on community health workers and local health centres rather than national hospitals. The World Bank has estimated that to provide clean water to all those in need would cost about $260 billion, which, although a vast sum, is only about half of one year's global expenditure on military arms.

Medicine is unavoidably concerned with the rational distribution of scarce resources, and as such it necessarily involves making political and economic decisions on the allocation of those resources. This is a particularly important issue in a poor country, where the cost of waste is so much greater than it is in a rich one.

The importance of education in improving the health of the world cannot be overestimated. Much of the difficulty in the introduction of measures designed to improve health is due to cultural or religious obstacles. Such obstacles to health may take the form of traditional practices that are deeply ingrained. In a poor country, people attempt to obtain long-term security by having large families, so that birth control, while of benefit to the community, may not be attractive to the individual. Social and cultural changes must progress together with economic development in a way that is sensitive and responsive to all the relevant issues. Few would doubt that the rich industrialised countries of the world have an obligation to provide a lead – but to be effective, they will need to recognise the cultural and political obstacles to prevention as well as the economic ones.

Glossary

The **absolute excess risk** of a disease in relation to a particular exposure is the incidence of the disease among exposed persons minus the incidence among non-exposed persons. (In this sense 'exposed' is used loosely to include having a 'factor', such as high blood pressure, compared to not having it, and so being 'unexposed'.)

The **attributable proportion** or **attributable fraction** is the proportion of cases of a disease that can be attributed to an exposure.

A **case–control study** is an observational study in which a group of individuals who have a particular disease or disorder (cases), and another group who do not (controls) are asked about or tested for the factor being studied, e.g. persons with and without lung cancer asked about their past smoking habits.

A **cause** of a disease is a factor that is associated with the disease so that if the intensity or frequency of exposure to the factor in a population is changed, the frequency of the disease also changes.

A **cohort study** is an observational study in which first an exposure or factor is estimated (by measurement or enquiry) in a group of individuals, and then the cause-specific disease incidence (or mortality) is recorded after a period of follow-up, e.g. the smoking habits of persons recorded and the subsequent incidence of lung cancer recorded on smokers and non-smokers. A cohort study can also be called a 'prospective' or 'longitudinal' study.

A **confounding factor** is a factor that explains, entirely or in part, an observed association between a study factor and a disease because of its association with both the study factor and the disease.

Confidence intervals indicate the range of values that is likely to include the true value. So the statement 'the 95% confidence interval is from 10 to 14' means that we can be 95% certain that the true value will lie within the interval 10–14 (inclusive). The meaning of '95% certain' is that if the same study were repeated 100 times, in 95 the confidence interval would include the true value but in 5 it would not.

The **detection rate** (**DR**) or **sensitivity** of a test is the proportion of affected individuals with positive test results.

A **double-blind** trial is one in which neither the patient nor the observer knows to which of the treatment regimens any patient in the trial is allocated. This is usually achieved by using a placebo.

Epidemiology is the study of the incidence, distribution and determinants of diseases in human populations with a view to identifying their causes and bringing about their prevention.

Error can be random or systematic. See entry under 'imprecision' for the former, and entry under 'systematic error' for the latter. Figure 1 on page 4 illustrates the two types of error.

The **false-positive rate (FPR)** of a test is the proportion of unaffected individuals with positive test results.

A **geographical control group** is a control group of patients with the same disorder as the cases but situated in a different place, say another hospital. Bias can be introduced by using a geographical control group.

A **historical control group** is a control group of patients with the same disorder as the cases but seen in the past. Bias can be introduced by using a historical control group.

Imprecision (random error) is poor repeatability, regardless of whether the results are, on average, accurate (see Figure 1 on page 4).

The **incidence** of a disease is the number of new cases that occur in a defined population in a specified period of time.

An **intention-to-treat** analysis is an analysis that includes all the persons randomised into a clinical trial, whether or not they complied with, or completed, the regimen under study. The analysis is carried out according to the group to which they were randomised and not according to whether the treatment or intervention was received.

Lead time bias is the time by which the diagnosis of a cancer is advanced by early detection without changing the date of death.

Length time bias is the apparent increase in survival due to the tendency to selectively detect slowly growing cancers instead of typical cancers.

A **longitudinal study** is the same as a cohort or prospective study.

A **nested case–control study** is a study in which the cases and a matched sample of controls are identified from a cohort study and data of aetiological interest applicable to when the cohort was recruited are obtained and compared in the cases and controls.

The **odds of being affected given a positive result (OAPR)** is the ratio of the number of affected to unaffected individuals among those with positive test results.

Precision is good repeatability (see Figure 1 on page 4).

The **positive predictive value** is the odds of being affected given a positive result expressed as a proportion or percentage.

The **prevalence** of a disease is the number of cases of a disease present in a defined population at a given point in time.

Primary prevention is the prevention of new cases of a disease by removing a cause of the disease.

A **prospective study** is the same as a cohort study. A nested case–control study is also prospective. It is not necessary to describe clinical or prevention trials as prospective.

The *p*-**value** is the probability that an observed difference between two population samples or one that is more extreme arose by chance, i.e. when there is, in fact, no difference between the two populations in what is being measured.

Random error See entry under 'imprecision' and Figure 1 on page 4.

A **real association** is an association between a factor and a disease that is not due to chance. It will then be either causal or due to bias or confounding. (Sometimes the term is restricted to mean an association that is causal or due to confounding but not due to measurement bias.) An association is usually assumed to be real when it is statistically significant.

The **relative risk** of a disease in relation to a particular exposure is the incidence of the disease among exposed persons divided by the incidence of the disease among unexposed persons. (In this sense 'exposed' is used loosely to include having a 'factor', such as high blood pressure, compared to not having it, and so being 'unexposed'.)

A **retrospective study** is the same as a case–control study.

Screening is the systematic application of a test or inquiry, to identify individuals at sufficient risk of a specific disorder to benefit from further investigation or direct preventive action, among persons who have not sought medical attention on account of symptoms of that disorder.

Sensitivity See *detection rate*.

Secondary prevention is the prevention of overt (clinical) cases of a disease through screening and early detection followed by appropriate intervention. It is sometimes also used to mean the prevention of the recurrence of a clinical event, e.g. the secondary prevention of heart attacks can mean prevention of future heart attacks in persons who have already had one.

The **specificity** of a test is the complement of the false-positive rate, i.e. the false-positive rate, expressed as a percentage subtracted from 100.

The **standardised mortality ratio** (SMR) is the ratio of the observed number of deaths in a study population to the expected number of deaths (from applying rates in a standard population), multiplied by 100.

Systematic error is the same as bias (or inaccuracy), meaning not being on target regardless of whether the results are repeatable. See Figure 1 on page 4.

Tertiary prevention is clinical treatment of a disease that prevents disability and pain resulting from that disease.

List of abbreviations

AIDS   Acquired immune deficiency syndrome
COAD   Chronic obstructive airways (sometimes 'lung' or 'pulmonary') disease
CMO   Chief Medical Officer
DEFRA   Department of Environment, Food and Rural Affairs
DR   Detection rate
FPR   False-positive rate
GNP   Gross national product
HIV   Human immunodeficiency virus
IHD   Ischaemic heart disease
LR   Likelihood ratio
NS-SEC   National Statistics Socio-economic Classification
OAPR   Odds of being affected given a positive result
OHE   Office of Health Economics
ONS   Office of National Statistics (formerly called OPCS)
OPCS   Office of Population Censuses and Surveys
PHLS   Public Health Laboratory Service
RCT   Randomised controlled trial
RR   Relative risk
SMR   Standardised mortality ratio
WHO   World Health Organisation

Appendix I: Selected sources of statistics

There are numerous sources of health and related statistics, some well publicised and others obscure. Some of the more widely accessible are listed below. The Office for National Statistics (ONS) (formerly the Office of Population Censuses and Surveys, OPCS) publishes a wide range of data that in many instances are regularly updated and are often the definitive source. The annual reports are published about two years in arrears, but there is a quarterly journal of the ONS called *Population Trends* that has recent statistics and articles analysing them. Many data series from published reports are also posted on the web at http://www.statistics.gov.uk/statbase.

Useful ONS publications (w = available on the web site)

Series Title and type of data

w	AB	Legal abortions: by woman's age, area of residence, gestation, method
w	CEN	Census: 10-yearly on entire population. Limited data on chronic illness, housing, ethnic group, social class, occupation, car ownership as index of affluence, etc
w	DH1	Mortality statistics serial tables, general trends in cancer and in respiratory disease mortality
w	DH2	Mortality statistics: cause
w	DH3	Mortality statistics: childhood
	DH4	Mortality statistics: accidents/violence
	DH5	Mortality statistics: area
w	DS	Occupational mortality
	EL	Electoral statistics: parliamentary
w	FM1	Birth statistics: by maternal age, area of residence, place of delivery, multiple births
w	FM2	Marriage and divorce
w	GH2	General household series: see below
	LS	Longitudinal study: based on a random 1% of the population. Records deaths, births, infant mortality and cancer, and is correlated against data from Census
w	MB1	Cancer statistics: registration

w	MB2	Communicable disease statistics
	MB3	Congenital malformations
	MB4	Hospital in-patient enquiry (ended 1985)
	MB5	Morbidity Statistics from General Practice
w	M N	Migration
w	PP1	Provisional mid-year population estimates
w	PP2	Population projections: key features for England and Wales
	PP3	Population projections: regions, counties, metropolitan districts and London boroughs
w	SMDS	Mortality statistics: perinatal and infant
w	VS	Local authority vital statistics: live and stillbirths, and death registrations
	WR	Registrar General's weekly return

Health Surveys for England

http://www.statistics.gov.uk/statbase

Carried out annually since 1990.

Living in Britain (formerly called General Household Survey)

http://www.statistics.gov.uk/statbase

Carried out annually on a stratified random sample of 12 500 with a response rate of 84%. Questions vary from year to year, but might cover:

- Health issues: smoking, alcohol, chronic illness or disability that limits activity, acute illness, GP consultation, hospital admission, contraception, dental health, accidents at home, glasses or contact lenses, health of elderly people.
- Social issues: leisure, housing, marriage, fertility, family education, employment, ethnic group.

Department of Health, Hospital Episode Statistics

This is a record of all hospital admissions, completed after discharge or death; it records principal diagnoses by age, sex, duration of admission, speciality, hospital, area of residence, health district and region.

Social Trends

http://www.statistics.gov.uk/statbase

Published by the Government Statistical Office; reports data from various government departments and special attitude surveys on numerous health and social issues.

Morbidity Statistics from General Practice

OPCS Series MB5

Forty 'Sentinel' general practices throughout Britain record details of all general practice consultations and hospital referrals by age, sex and principal diagnoses.

World Health Statistics

http://www.who.int/

Published annually by the World Health Organisation; gives data of births, deaths, infant mortality, cause of death, etc. for most countries.

World Development Report

http://www.worldbank.org/

Published annually by Oxford University Press for the World Bank. Includes many economic indicators and development indicators such as birth rate, death rate, infant mortality, use of contraception, life expectancy, health expenditure, fertility and nutrition.

Compendium of Health Statistics

http://www.ohe.org/

Published by the Office of Health Economics; 9th edition in 1995. Gives population and vital statistics and UK health care expenditure in detail.

The National Food Survey

http://www.statistics.gov.uk/statbase

The Department of Environment, Food and Rural Affairs (DEFRA) surveys 8000 households annually. Over a 7-day period, all food purchased for consumption is recorded. Mean values of energy, protein, carbohydrate, fat, vitamin and mineral intake are calculated.

Appendix II: Death certificates

Statement of cause of death

The details of cause of death in a death certificate provide information of great use to epidemiologists. They can be used to quantify the variation of fatal disease with age, sex, locality, occupation or medical history. When special measures have been taken to prevent or cure a particular condition, the statistics will assist the monitoring of the programme – for example, trends in death from cervical cancer. To illustrate how these figures come about, the following is an extract from the notes for medical practitioners when completing a death certificate in *Forms for Medical Certificates of the Cause of Death*.

The concept of the underlying cause of death

Since certification began in Britain, the national statistics have been based on what is referred to as the 'Underlying Cause of Death' – that is the disease or injury that initiated the train of morbid events leading to death. The certificate is laid out so that several conditions can be set out in a sequence. When more than one condition is to be recorded, the most recent should be inserted in Ia. The disease or antecedent cause that led to this should be inserted in Ib (and similarly for Ic, if appropriate). This provides the certifier with the opportunity to set out the main disease processes that have affected the deceased. The Underlying Cause of Death, i.e. that which initiated the train of events leading ultimately to death, should appear in the lowest completed line of Part I of the certificate. However, there is no need to record the mode of dying (such as heart failure or asphyxia). Addition of a statement of the mode of dying does not assist in deriving mortality statistics, when the underlying cause of death is explicitly stated (e.g. cardiac arrest following myocardial infarction). Even more important is the need to avoid completing a certificate with the mode of dying as the only entry; this should be the subject of further enquiry if the disease process involved is genuinely not known. Many patients with major disease may develop a 'terminal bronchopneumonia'; again, there is no need to record this final event in the sequence. Because the main statistics are based on coding of the Underlying Cause of Death, it is essential that the certificate sets out clearly the major disease involved – such as the specific cancer, ischaemic heart disease or chronic bronchitis. For example:

I	(a)	Cerebral metastases	3 weeks
	(b)	Primary bronchial carcinoma	2 years
	(c)	—	
II		—	

Handling multiple pathology

When there is a major disease present, plus some other quite different diseases *that contribute to death*, but are not part of the sequence of stages of the major disease (such as chronic bronchitis in a patient with advanced atherosclerotic disease), the second disease should be recorded in Part II of the certificate. For example:

I	(a)	Myocardial infarction	7 days
	(b)	Coronary atheroma	4 years
	(c)	—	
II		Chronic bronchitis	11 years

Part II should not be used to list all the diseases present at death (for example, in the elderly), unless there is difficulty in deciding whether the presence of each of the additional conditions hastened the death of the patient.

Rather different are the more complicated situations when there are two (or more) major and distinct diseases present, and it is difficult to identify which of the two conditions was the one that led to death. The current death certificate is not ideally suited to recording such multiple pathology. For example, with an elderly person suffering from manifestations of coronory artery disease, and also chronic bronchitis, the clinician may conclude that these jointly led to death (or he may even consider it inappropriate to identify only one of the two as the main cause of death). Both conditions should then be inserted in Part I of the certificate, and an annotation inserted to indicate that death was due to a combination of the two diseases. For example:

I	(a)	Coronary atheroma and Chronic bronchitis (joint causes of death)

With such a certificate, the coders will invoke an arbitrary rule that selects one cause for the underlying cause. In some elderly persons, there may be no specific condition identified as the patient gradually fails. If such circumstances gradually lead to deterioration and ultimate death then 'old age' or 'senility' is perfectly acceptable as the sole cause of death for persons aged 70 and over.

Specificity

The value of the information is enhanced when the statement of the cause of death is as specific as possible – for example carcinoma of the ascending colon (rather than malignant tumour of the bowel), acute monocytic leukaemia (rather than leukaemia) or chronic glomerulonephritis (rather than renal failure). When known, the duration between onset and death should be recorded, as this may affect the coding of the cause of death (particularly when late effects are distinguished). For example:

I	(a)	Cor pulmonale	6 weeks
	(b)	Pulmonary fibrosis	14 years
	(c)	Inactive pulmonary tuberculosis	26 years
II		Peptic ulcer	6 years

This would be coded to 'late effects of respiratory tuberculosis'.

When appropriate, information should be given about operations or drugs that may have led to adverse effects.

MED A
14

Register to enter
No. of Death Entry

000000

BIRTHS AND DEATHS REGISTRATION ACT 1953

(Form prescribed by the Registration of Births, Deaths and Marriages (Amendment) Regulations 1985)

MEDICAL CERTIFICATE OF CAUSE OF DEATH

For use only by a Registered Medical Practitioner WHO HAS BEEN IN ATTENDANCE during the deceased's last illness,
and to be delivered by him forthwith to the Registrar of Births and Deaths.

Name of deceased ....

Date of death as stated to me .... day of .... 19 ......   Age as stated to me ....

Place of death ....

Last seen alive by me .... day of .... 19 ......

1 The certified cause of death takes account of information obtained from post-mortem.

2 Information from post-mortem may be available later.

3 Post-mortem not being held.

4 I have reported this death to the Coroner for further action.
   [See overleaf]

Please ring appropriate digit(s) and letter.

a Seen after death by me.

b Seen after death by another medical practitioner but not by me.

c Not seen after death by a medical practitioner.

CAUSE OF DEATH

The condition thought to be the 'Underlying Cause of Death' should appear in the lowest completed line of Part I

I(a) Disease or condition directly leading to death† ....

(b) Other disease or condition, if any, leading to I(a) ....

(c) Other disease or condition, if any, leading to I(b) ....

II Other significant conditions CONTRIBUTING TO THE DEATH but not related to the disease or condition causing it. ....

These particulars not to be entered in death register

Approximate interval between onset and death

The death might have been due to or contributed to by the employment followed at some time by the deceased. ....

Please tick where applicable

†*This does not mean the mode of dying, such as heart failure, asphyxia, asthenia, etc: it means the disease, injury, or complication which caused death.*

I hereby certify that I was in medical attendance during the above named deceased's last illness, and that the particulars and cause of death above written are true to the best of my knowledge and belief.

Signature ....

Residence ....

Qualifications as registered by General Medical Council

Date ....

For deaths in hospital: Please give the name of the consultant responsible for the above-named as a patient. ....

Complete where applicable

A	B
I have reported this death to the Coroner for further action.	I may be in a position later to give, on application by the Registrar General, additional information as to the cause of death for the purpose of more precise statistical classification.
Initials of certifying medical practitioner.	Initials of certifying medical practitioner. ....

The Coroner needs to consider all cases where:

    The death might have been due to or contributed to by a violent or unnatural cause (including an accident);

or the cause of death cannot be identified;

or the death might have been due to or contributed to by drugs, medicine, abortion or poison;

or there is reason to believe that the death occurred during an operation or under or prior to complete recovery from an anaesthetic or arising subsequently out of an incident during an operation or an anaesthetic;

or the death might have been due to or contributed to by the employment followed at some time by the deceased.

LIST OF SOME OF THE CATEGORIES OF DEATH WHICH MAY BE OF INDUSTRIAL ORIGIN

MALIGNANT DISEASES — Causes include:

(a) Skin
- radiation and sunlight
- pitch or tar
- mineral oils

(b) Nasal
- wood or leather work
- nickel

(c) Lung
- asbestos
- nickel
- radiation

(d) Pleura
- asbestos

(e) Urinary Tract
- benzidine
- dyestuff
- chemicals in rubbers

(f) Liver
- PVC manufacture

(g) Bone
- radiation

(h) Lymphatics and haematopoietic
- radiation
- benzene

POISONING

(a) Metals e.g. arsenics, cadmium, lead

(b) Chemicals e.g. chlorine, benzene

(c) Solvents e.g. trichlorethylene

INFECTIOUS DISEASES — Causes include:

(a) Anthrax
- imported bone, bonemeal, hide or fur

(b) Brucellosis
- farming or veterinary

(c) Tuberculosis
- contact at work

(d) Leptospirosis
- farming, sewer or underground workers

(e) Tetanus
- farming or gardening

(f) Rabies
- animal handling

(g) Viral hepatitis
- contact at work

BRONCHIAL ASTHMA AND PNEUMONITIS

(a) Occupational asthma
- sensitising agent at work

(b) Allergic Alveolitis
- farming

PNEUMOCONIOSIS
- mining and quarrying
- potteries
- asbestos

NOTE:—The Practitioner, on signing the certificate, should complete, sign and date the Notice to the Informant, which should be detached and handed to the Informant. The Practitioner should then, without delay, deliver the certificate itself to the Registrar of Births and Deaths for the sub-district in which the death occurred. Envelopes for enclosing the certificates are supplied by the Registrar.

Appendix III: Conceptual similarity between statistical significance testing and screening

A p-value is analogous to a false-positive rate as used in screening terminology. For example, $p \leq 0.05$ (or $\leq 5\%$) is equivalent to a 5% false-positive rate. It indicates that when there is no true difference between the groups being compared, a positive result (one with a difference as large as or larger than the one observed) will occur by chance in 5% of such studies, so it is, in a sense, a false-positive. Such a 'positive' result is said to be one that is statistically significant.

The statistical power of a study is analogous to the detection rate as used in screening terminology. It indicates the probability that a particular study will yield a positive (statistically significant) result when one, of a specified magnitude or greater, genuinely exists.

Using the screening analogy, if a study has an 80% power of detecting a difference at a p-value of 0.05, the study has an 80% chance of detecting a true-positive and a $\leq 5\%$ chance of producing a false-positive. In screening, detection and false-positive rates apply to tests performed on affected and unaffected individuals. In statistics, the corresponding terms, statistical power and p-value, apply to studies carried out on different samples of individuals in which, for example, the means of the variable of interest are compared to see if they are different in the populations from which the samples were taken. (The section on screening that you may want to refer to is on page 30.) The table on the next page illustrates the conceptual similarity between a screening test and statistical significance testing.

Screening test	Statistical significance testing
Aim Method to distinguish affected from unaffected individuals	**Aim** Method to determine whether there is a genuine difference in a variable between two groups by comparing samples from each group
Cut-off Value of the screening variable that defines a positive test	**Critical difference** Difference that is important enough to detect
Detection rate Proportion of *affected* individuals with positive results	**Power of the study** Proportion of times such a study will give a positive (i.e. statistically significant) result when there is a difference at least as great as the critical difference
False-positive rate Proportion of *unaffected* individuals with positive results	**p-value** Proportion of times a study will, on average, give a positive result when there is no difference
To improve discrimination Increase detection rate for a given false-positive rate, i.e. find a more discriminatory screening test or combine several tests so that the overlap in the screening variable between affected and unaffected is reduced	**To increase power of study for a given p-value** Increase sample size of study. The means from large samples have a tighter spread (less random variation) than the spread of means from small samples. A difference as large as or larger than the critical difference is then less likely to arise by chance

References and further reading

Books and journal articles

Ahlbom A, Norell S. *Introduction to Modern Epidemiology*. Chestnut Hill, MA: Epidemiology Resources Inc, 1990.

Donaldson L. *CMO's Update 33*. London: Department of Health, 2002.

Friedman GD. *Primer of Epidemiology*, 4th edn. New York: McGraw Hill, 1994.

Hill AB. *Principles of Medical Statistics*, 12th edn. London: Edward Arnold, 1991.

ISIS. Randomised trial of intravenous streptokinase, oral aspirin, both, or neither among 17,187 cases of suspected acute myocardial infarction: ISIS-2. *Lancet* 1988; **ii**: 349–59.

King MH. Medicine in an unjust world. In: Weatherall DJ, Ledingham JGG, Warrell DA (eds). *Oxford Textbook of Medicine*, Vol 1. Oxford: Oxford University Press, 1983: 3.3–3.11.

Law MR, Wald NJ, Thompson SG. By how much and how quickly does reduction in serum cholesterol concentration lower risk of ischaemic heart disease? *Br Med J* 1994; **308**: 367–72.

Law MR, Wald NJ. Risk factor thresholds: their existence under scrutiny. *Br Med J* 2003; **324**: 1570–6.

McKeown T. *The Role of Medicine*. Oxford: Blackwell, 1984.

Rohan TE, Frost CD, Wald NJ. Prevention of blindness by screening for diabetic retinopathy: a quantitative assessment. *Br Med J* 1989; **299**: 1198–201.

Rose G. *The Strategy of Preventive Medicine*. Oxford: Oxford University Press, 1992.

Wald NJ, Leck I (eds). *Antenatal and Neonatal Screening*, 2nd edn. Oxford: Oxford University Press, 2000.

Wald N, Boreham J, Bailey A. Serum retinol and subsequent risk of cancer. *Br J Cancer* 1986; **54**: 957–61.

Web sites

Centers for Disease Control & Prevention (CDC)
http://www.cdc.gov/
CDC is one of the best sites for information on chronic diseases and injuries. This site also provides full text access to the *Morbidity and Mortality Weekly Reports.*

National Institutes of Health
http://www.nih.gov/

National Library of Medicine
http://www.nlm.nih.gov/

The Cochrane Collaboration
http://www.cochrane.org

Index